I can't let you disappear in death, the way you disappeared in life. That's why I'm here, breaking my heart all over again.

BEFORE I GROW OLD

LINDA RUTH BROOKS

...a memoir for my son...

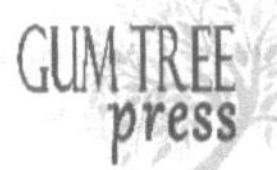

GUM TREE
press

A catalogue record for this book is available from the National Library of Australia

Cover, text design, typesetting & interior design by *Linda Ruth Brooks*
Photo artwork: *Linda Ruth Brooks*

ISBN: 978-1-7644921-6-4: 9798257378966

Before I grow old: memoir for my son…, and other books by Linda Brooks may be purchased through online bookstores and retail outlets

Author

Linda Brooks lives in Adelaide. She writes nonfiction, poetry, fiction and short stories. She has published and illustrated children's books. She is a Rebecca Coyle Scholar and has a BA Hons in Creative Writing from Southern Cross University.

She gained a publisher for her childhood memoir *A Curious & Inelegant Childhood*. She has written a nonfiction book on living with Asperger's Syndrome *I'm not broken, I'm just different* and the children's book *Callan the Chameleon* with contributions from Professor Tony Attwood.

Published in anthologies: Coastlines 5, 6, 7 & 8 (Southern Cross University); 'Wood, Bricks & Stone – the Making of the Hunter' (Catchfire Press); 'Grieve' (Hunter Writer's Centre); 'Third Wednesday Poets' (TWP); 'Longing for Solitude' (Central Coast Poets); 'The Great Escape' (Newcastle Herald); 'A Far Place' (Stringybark Press); 'Space in a Time of COVID'.

Awards: First prize for The Legacy University Level Creative Writing Award; first prize in the Gabe Reynaud Creative Writing Award, the Mater Misericordiae Grieve Writing Award and the Rebecca Coyle Scholarship for BA Hons.

A registered nurse and advocate for disability in a previous life, Linda has a rich background in listening to the stories of others, never shying away from the darker, gritty tales. And yet, humour is never far away. Linda enjoys hearing from her readers (even if they've found typos):
    lindaruthbrooks@bigpond.com

Author titles

Nonfiction:
I'm not broken, I'm just different
(on autism with Professor Tony Attwood)
A Curious and Inelegant Childhood

Poetry:
The Long Acre Paddock
Verse

Fiction:
A broken hallelujah
Behind Whispering Hands
Butterfly Pinning
Prose: stuff I never told you
Scarlett doesn't live here anymore
The Lost stories of Lucy Meredith Carter
The Unprize
Under the Bracken Fern

Publisher of the anthologies:
We are Australian
The Great Australian Shed
Waltzing Matilda

Children's books:
A Tabby Never Forgets
Callan the Chameleon
Dusty Bunny's Very Important Job
Izzy & Pudding the Cat
I want a monkey!
Madam Iris Bigglesworth
The Banyula Tales - 6 stories
Who Stole Christmas?

Author's Note

Any likeness to any person living or dead is quite possibly intentional and you should probably take a good hard look at yourself—like I did; and it wasn't easy. I changed most of the names to protect anyone and everyone, but especially my sons. Perhaps, I should have changed them to protect the innocent, or maybe the guilty. Anyway, I couldn't work out who was which; the guilty or the innocent. Life isn't always about guilt or innocence, for we all share the fabric of life, this wonderful, fragile, flawed cloak of humanity. I am no longer afraid of being guilty or innocent. For I am human. And I am both.

In order to give an authentic view of Gerard's life and struggles, I have written about his father and stepfather, and their impact on him. This is not always a flattering view, so I feel constrained to include only those events that affected Gerard.

After all, it's only fair, as I have studiously omitted some of my own crimes and misdemeanours.

The only truly innocent in the story is Mr Clooney, the ginger cat, who, as we speak, is nibbling my foot as if it were a ham sandwich because I annoyed him by patting his paw the wrong way. He features not only as an integral part but also because Gerard took me to the animal rescue place, where Mr Clooney instantly chose me by climbing a stick and purring a clear 'take me!'

I admit it's impossible to write a single word about a life with accuracy. Every memory is a half-remembered thing. And anyone in any family can attest that everyone has a different story about events shared with siblings or parents. Trauma increases the distance between the narratives we tell.

This is Gerard's story, and inevitably that means it is also my story.

A note

Trigger warning.
Readers are advised that this book contains references to
potentially distressing topics, including suicide and family
violence.

Contents

Arrival

'Nurse! Nurse! Get moving!'

The midwife's voice rose, penetrating the fog, jerking me into belated action. Towels, towels! I ran for the warm towels. Another babe had entered the world, pink, squirming and miraculous, leaving me in dreamlike awe, instead of a functioning nurse trainee assisting in a birth. It got me every time. The wonder. The sheer power of a life arriving. One person becoming two.

Shaken out of my reverie, I made myself useful. I'd been on the Maternity Ward for a month and knew the drill, but the babies, those marvellous new humans, how they enchanted me.

Naturally, it was less exciting in those nursery times when 21 or more infants all cried at once, setting each other off in a cacophony of warbling. Yet to have a baby in my arms. It fulfilled in a way nothing else did.

A year later, a nurse wheeled me down the hall and into a labour ward. My huge watermelon belly rolled uncomfortably. I had waited for this day. Planned for it. Knitted and crocheted for it.

Having been a trainee at the same hospital, I knew the wards, knew the staff, and they knew me. I was met with knowing grins.

'How are you doing, Brooks?' the Sister asked, hands on hips.

'I've changed my mind,' I said, fear of the unknown settling in, 'I want to go home. This is all a mistake. This,' I said, patting my stomach, 'is just a big lunch.'

The Sister laughed, flicked surgical gloves on with a slap – a sound I had previously enjoyed but now seemed ominous.

'Are you going to be trouble, Brooks?' she asked.

A nurse in the corner giggled.

'I see my reputation precedes me,' I said haughtily. 'I can't promise anything.'

Another snapping of gloves. The obstetrician arrived. Induction of labour at 8:30 am for a recalcitrant babe that was nearly three weeks late and showing no inclination to join the world. A foreboding of a life to come.

Hoisted into the stirrups and surrounded by white uniforms, gowns and masks, I closed my eyes. For the first time, there was no need for me to be alert.

'The cervix has no feeling,' said the doctor, as a metallic crunch signalled the clamping of my cervix.

'Who the hell told you that?' I shrieked, 'A man?'

He smiled, gave instructions for copious drugs and left the fray.

Labour was immediate and intense. Before he even left the hospital, I was having fierce contractions every few minutes.

With every contraction, the mask was shoved on my face.

'Stop that, you girls!' I said, tugging at the mask. 'You're only doing this to shut me up. That bloody mask isn't making any difference. I can't breathe with that thing on my face!'

In the following hours, I broke every rule, grabbed the top of the iron bed, rambled, yowled and told stories, barely aware of my words or actions, as I was administered Pethidine regularly without asking. I talked complete rubbish. Grabbed my husband, Guy's arm, refusing to let him leave the room even for the loo. Apparently, I gave instructions to everyone in the room. I remembered very little of it, and when Guy relayed my nonsense back the following day, I found out the hard way that laughing hurt more than crying after a caesarean section.

I was so wasted that I could only keep one eye open at a time. I remember badgering the staff for updates. I squinted at the clock. I kept one blurry eye on proceedings, not registering much and completely unaware of how much free entertainment I was providing the staff. I stared out of the second-floor window and swore blind I had washing on the line that I needed to bring in immediately. I argued about having buns in the oven that would burn. (I had recently been trying my hand at breadmaking).

Then, for my pièce de résistance, I took over the whole show. I scowled at the clock and, through my dozy haze, realised with clarity that I had been pushing in the "last stage of labour" for five hours. I heard the midwifery Sister ask for forceps, heard the clatter of instruments, the hurried movements, the silence, the trolley wheels…

Concentrating with great difficulty, I unhooked my legs from the stirrups, one at a time.

'No. No, no,' I said, 'that's not happening. I've been pushing with everything I have for five hours, fully dilated, and if this baby hasn't arrived through the birth canal, then it's not meant to come that way. Get the doctor. Get an anaesthetist. Get the theatre and get me out of here!'

To show I meant business, I crossed my legs. No small feat.

I must have convinced them because some time later, I was being transferred to the theatre. Once wheeled into the operating room and placed on the table, I continued my one-eyed surveillance. Watching the white-gowned, masked staff, I worked out which one was the anaesthetist, grabbed his coat and yanked hard. He jumped. 'Will you, for crying out loud, put me to sleep already?' I said.

'Oh, I can't just yet,' he said reasonably, trying to free himself from my grip. 'We have to wait for the surgeon. But you can stop pushing now, dear.'

'Easy for you to say,' I muttered.

At 2 am, still desperately dopey, when the nurses wheeled me from the Recovery Ward and headed to the Maternity Ward, I rebelled. Quietly. I desperately wanted to see my new son. I hadn't known his gender before. A son. I'd had a general anaesthetic due to the emergency status, so there had been no wondrous union with my babe on my chest. I hadn't seen him. I was told that he was 8 lbs 10 in the old money. A whopper. The biggest of the newborns. Later, I was told that preliminary X-rays showed a risk for natural delivery due to a small pelvis.

At the lift to go down a floor to the patient rooms, I put both arms out so they couldn't get me into the lift. I protested that I wasn't going anywhere until I'd seen my son. It was impossible, they said. I told them what rubbish that was and that they could wheel me past the nursery window and hold him up. But, they said, 'he's in the infrared crib. He was a bit jaundiced. It's not possible.'

'Then just wheel me past,' I begged, my voice groggy but plaintive. 'Just a little peek. Please. I know I can't touch him, hold him, but surely I can see him.'

They exchanged glances, smiled and nodded.

I squinted with one eye, then another, as my son was brought to the nursery window. I cried with relief, called him beautiful, pointed to his big head, and those lovely nurses didn't tell me that I was looking at the wrong end.

Birth Registry

Here's some advice you never knew you needed. Don't send a dyslexic to the Birth Registry.

When I was pregnant with Gerard, my first husband, Guy, and I discussed prospective baby names at a family event. It was kind of cool having input from relatives about names. I loved the name Lincoln. I was determined not to name a child after some long-dead relative I had never met. Guy had a host of those. I would have liked Lincoln Max, but one must compromise. There were a lot of Jarred's with various spellings. There was an ad on the telly with a nerdy bloke named Gerrard, with slow emphasis on the last syllable, GerrARD. I wanted to avoid that. I did, however, like the French spelling and pronunciation. We scribbled names to see what we thought and decided on Gerard. At least that's what I thought.

However, when Gerard was born, I was incapacitated after a C-section, so I had to leave the paperwork to Guy. I don't trust anyone else with paperwork. I'm fussy. I'm the only one who will get it right. I filled in my parents' forms all the time. My mother wouldn't tick the widow box after Dad died because she still loved him and refused to disconnect in any way. So I looked forward to the birth forms and was disappointed when I had to leave them to Guy.

Off I went into life with "Gerard", never thinking of GerrARD, never suspecting that he had been registered as GerrARD by his Dyslexic father. We didn't know of Guy's dyslexia at the time. This delusion went on for years for me. You might question my sanity at this point, but it was the eighties. You could open a bank account without an ID, and you could enrol your child in any number of places with no verification of their identity at all. You could go off to doctors' surgeries, preschool, school and not need a birth certificate. When it came to Centrelink and parenting payments, I used the Gerard spelling with no problem. At school, he was Gerard. All his books and possessions were written that way.

Gerard's father didn't notice. Guy never filled in a form while I knew him, in the four years we were married. He never wrote Gerard's name, and then he legged it to America after the divorce and never wrote a letter to his son.

Contact was minimal. Guy kept his whereabouts secret to avoid paying child support, so there were only occasional phone calls. I corresponded with Guy's parents—Gerard's grandparents.

Gerard's bank account was in the name of Gerard.

You can see a clear prejudice here. Held by me. He wasn't GerrARD, he was Gerard.

Guy returned to Australia for his grandmother, Ruby's 100th birthday. Gerard's wedding was happening the day after the birthday celebrations. Then it was "GerrARD this" and "GerrARD that" on the invitations and marriage forms, which I took personally. This was wrong!

To make matters worse, Gerard adopted the GerrARD spelling after a lifetime of being Gerard. He said GerrARD was on his birth certificate. I wondered why I didn't have said birth certificate. Clearly a monumental error on my part, not possessing a birth certificate for my child. No one produced a birth certificate. He was married as GerrARD. I couldn't get a birth certificate for an adult child. At least that's what the registry told me.

When Gerard returned to live with me in 2016, it was still niggling my poor brain. In my mind, I had been lied to.

Gerard didn't have any of his documents in paper form, so we applied for a copy of his birth certificate. I waited for it to arrive so I could prove this terrible lie.

I tore the letter open when it arrived. I was gobsmacked. According to the registry, my son's name was GerrARD.

I immediately rambled on to Gerard with the whole, complicated story.

'I thought you were lying, Gerard.'

'Silly little mother,' he said, rubbing the top of my head, a favourite habit. 'I get called Jared, GerrARD and all kinds of things, and it's never bothered me.

'I noticed that,' I said. 'You never correct anyone.'

He smiled.

'You'll always be Gerard to me.'

'I'm not filling in any more forms.'

So that's why you never send a dyslexic to the Birth Registry.

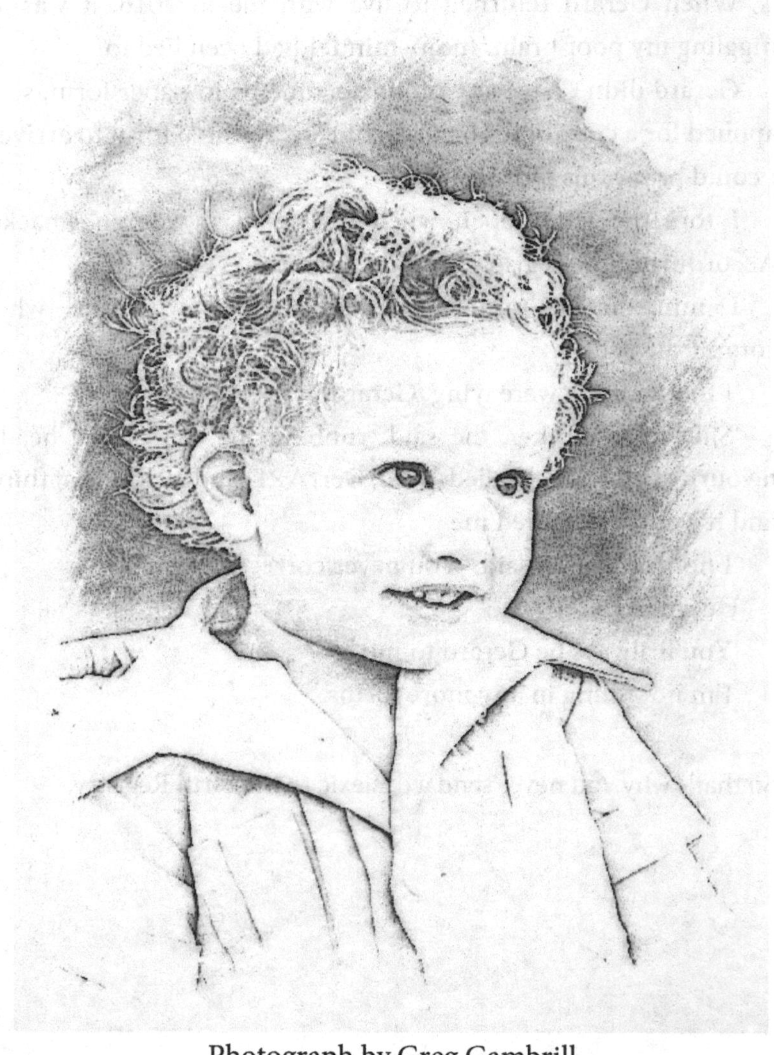

Photograph by Greg Gambrill

An autistic boy

Gerard was diagnosed as being on the autism spectrum at 36. The late diagnosis had a crushing effect on him. After his wife left him, he returned to live with me. He spoke of how differently he could have lived if he had known earlier. How much easier it would have been to advocate for an environment that didn't test his every nerve and push his limits.

While he was with me, I fought to get help for him in much the same way I had fought for his brother, Bronson. When Bronson moaned about having a book written about him, Gerard said, 'I wish it was my book.'

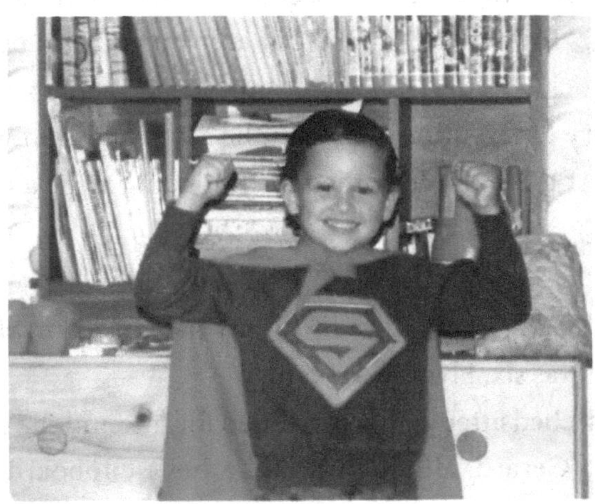

Gerard was eight when I took him to a professional clinical psychologist, Dr Greg Carter. It was a small clinic, or set of rooms, near the Newcastle Mater Hospital.

It wasn't the first time I sought help for my sombre little boy, so serious I wondered if he was depressed, then felt daft for thinking this of such a young child. But I had no better words for a boy who lived in his own world.

At four years of age, when people asked him what he was going to be when he grew up, he answered, 'I'm only four,' while looking at them as if they should know how unreasonable the question was. The audience response was inevitably surprised. They bent down, or squatted, in that manner of the adult addressing a child as a more immature being. They smiled, offered a few of the usual suspects: a train driver, a fireman.

Even the adults' bending-down pose and voice inflections seem to confuse Gerard. What was wrong with these people? However, if he were approached as if he were a short adult with the maturity and knowledge of an older person, he would answer with greater comfort.

The life destination question was particularly trying for him. It was nonsense. Adults never seemed to tire of it as a way of connecting. How old are you? What are you going to be when you grow up?

I had very different responses to the same question when asked as a child. At three, I told someone, 'I'm going to be a nurse and a typewriter.'

For Gerard's early years, I lived with my parents from when he was two until he was six. I had two rooms.

One was a bedsitter with a single bed for me, and the other room belonged to Gerard, although it had a huge cupboard where my mother kept her collections, her special interests. Many of which revolved around paper. Recycled gift paper that she had ironed after removing the sticky tape after receiving the paper as a gift.

However, whenever she wanted to wrap a present for someone, these meticulously preserved papers were rejected in favour of new wrapping paper, which was also in that cupboard and in generous supply. She had greeting cards, sympathy cards, thank-you cards, and birthday cards. All of which could be sourced at a moment's notice.

Gerard had a toy box, a pine wood box with a lid. Any of us putting anything on top of that toy box received a polite but firm reminder that the rule he mandated for the toy box was that nothing was ever to be placed on it. If his grandmother ever infringed the rule by temporarily placing any item, he would get her attention and say, 'Nana, what have I told you about my toy box?'

If he wanted to tell me something, he often approached it as if he were making an appointment. 'Mummy, I have something to tell you, and I would like you to sit down and listen, all right?'

The politeness of this approach and the mature sigh that went with it just broke me. I could never resist.

At five, he asked me to sit at the small table in the bedsit room. I was never sure if he was going to tell me something of great importance or if it was a minor matter, until I realised that all these conversations were of great importance to him. He already had the vocabulary of a high school student.

'Mummy,' he began, once I was seated in the correct chair, in the right way, which meant not half on the chair as if seeking imminent escape or partial engagement in the conversation. 'Mummy, I don't like being asked what I want to do when I grow up. But I will tell you. I want to be a father. I can't wait until I have a wife and children of my own.'

I was shocked. I wondered where this desire was coming from. Was it due to the divorce? The absence of his father? The knowledge that he had once had a baby brother?

As usual, I was probably off the mark completely. A child with autistic thought is often misunderstood, and I'm the first to admit I didn't have a clue.

'Oh,' I said. 'Where will you live?' As the question left my mouth, I felt it was a dumb thing to say.

'With you,' he said, 'of course.'

'How do you think your wife will feel about that? She mightn't agree.'

'I won't marry anyone that doesn't agree,' he said, with the kind of confident, matter-of-fact attitude usually found in politicians and not in small boys, and definitely not in his mother, ever.

As he got older, Gerard refused to answer the "what are you going to be" question. In fact, throughout life, he continued this practice with any and all questions, often with a small smile as if you should know better than to ask silly questions.

There was a superhero dress-up day at school, and I asked who he wanted to be. Superman. So I worked on a costume with his detailed instructions. It was imperative that his curly blonde hair was at least flattened. Superman did not have curls. Gerard wished he did not have curls. I took a photo. It was the only photo I ever took where Gerard posed for it. All other photos were impromptu.

I asked him what superpower he would like to have. Speed like Superman? Strength? flight?'

'Invisible,' he said, 'I'd like to be invisible.'

Before the beginning...

To know someone is to know their ancestors. Here are some of Gerard's.

There are others, but they all died of perfection, and perfection is profoundly boring.

Gerard's father

> This is where a picture of Gerard's father belongs, but I don't have permission so you will just have to use your imagination.

Winter-frosted grass crunched underfoot as I crossed the lawn in front of our house. I was sixteen. I sighed softly and shifted the heavy case of books from my right hand to my left. Not wishing to miss the school bus, I quickened my steps. In year 9, I no longer rode my pushbike. The bus was preferable to walking the three miles to school.

Our small country school was meeting with a posh Sydney school for our annual Swimming Carnival at a swanky city pool. This meant a long, hot train journey to the city for us country kids. By the time we arrived at the swimming pool, I was tired.

On the benches beside the pool, it was unbearably hot. I was annoyed that only competitors were allowed in the pool until all the races were over, allowing a meagre few minutes of cool relief for the rest of us before marching off to catch the train home. There was not even a faint hope that our school would win. We never did. After all, we had only ever swum in the local creek, where black factory sludge was deposited.

Guy, Gerard's father, was seventeen and a student at the city school. He had won several races that day. He stretched and curved his lithe frame at the edge of the pool while his current adoring girlfriend waited and held his towel.

There was a brief intermission between races. The tantalising nearness of the pool proved too much for me. I slipped into a corner of the pool, dipping below the delicious water, enjoying the cool slickness on my skin. When the starter gun fired for the next race, I climbed out of the side, bumping into Guy as he shook water from his curly hair. I muttered, 'bloody city snobs' and headed for the stands, receiving a barbed reprimand from a sunburnt teacher.

That might have been it for Guy and me, except for his family's relocation to the village where I lived.

I met Guy at church, on a glowing summer day, in the shade of several Jacaranda trees that drifted mauve florets on those standing below. When introduced to the group outside the seminary chapel, Guy didn't acknowledge anyone, but stood staring gloomily into the distance. He gave all the appearance of being terminally bored and didn't speak to anyone he was introduced to.

On his arrival, Guy began an earnest cycle of girlfriends. He was seen walking the village paths and wooded lanes with them, then jettisoning them with the same ease with which he had acquired them. Guy joined our Year 11 class even though he was two years older.

I thought him arrogant, proud.

Everyone groaned at the English curriculum that included a Shakespearean play. There was little to love about Richard III. Shakespeare, with cunning wit, had written the character with evil running through his veins.

Our English teacher decided that students would read various parts to help us understand the play. He chose Guy for the part of Richard III and me for the hapless Lady Anne. He flipped open the play and randomly selected a scene. It was a crude scene. Guy silkily read the seductive lines. I was shocked as I found the page and the lewd words. My only consolation in that humiliating experience was that Lady Anne told him to go to hell.

The Shakespearean reading seemed to spark Guy's interest in me. He began a lusty pursuit, one that I rebuffed at every turn.

He sat beside me on the long school benches for lunch. I got up and walked away. He tried to engage me in conversation, usually with a crass opening remark. 'Hey Linda. Sexy shoes,' he said, leaning back nonchalantly on the railing of the upstairs balcony.

I fumed. 'Ah, yes,' I said. 'They're called Shin Kickers. Fancy a demonstration?'

Guy laughed, but flushed.

I wondered why he hadn't found a new female to walk the paths with, to attach to. I wished he would leave me alone and go back to recycling girls. His advances stung in their crude delivery, their disrespectful words. I called him Mr No Manners, arrogant prat. I told him to learn some grace.

For a year, his advances only yielded cold disdain from me.

Then his behaviour changed. He was quieter. He stayed in class rather than taking off whenever he liked. He spent longer on his books.

I was relieved that he was no longer approaching me with sly remarks. However, he still approached. He stepped aside to let me pass before him through doors. He handed me a pen silently when I needed one. He lit my Bunsen burner in Science when I shrank from the task. He picked up my heavy case of books and walked me to the bus. He said very little. He called me by my name instead of offering only crass words. He praised my work.

There were no more word battles or crude remarks, no whistles as I passed.

At the end of the year, there was a class picnic on the beach. I sat with the girls around a bonfire. Someone brought out a guitar, and we sang. We unwrapped and ate burgers packed for the occasion as the salt air caressed and the pink twilight sun sank low.

When we were leaving, Guy wasted no time in corralling me, walking the length of the beach with me on our return to the bus for the journey home.

I tolerated his presence, half-pleased, half-reluctant, not sensing that the words I heard, the influence over me that Guy was slowly weaving, would become the tragic mischief of my life's drama. He spoke softly of his vulnerability, his isolation, his angst at being painted as the family's black sheep because he was different, not fitting. He related beatings at home, attempts to run away, and harsh punishments meted out by his father.

These vulnerable admissions, delivered with quiet voice and deference, won my affections and my sympathies as my young heart set aside Guy's dark moods and wild actions.

We married in 1975, the year I graduated from nursing.

Gerard was born two years later.

Maternal grandparents

Pa

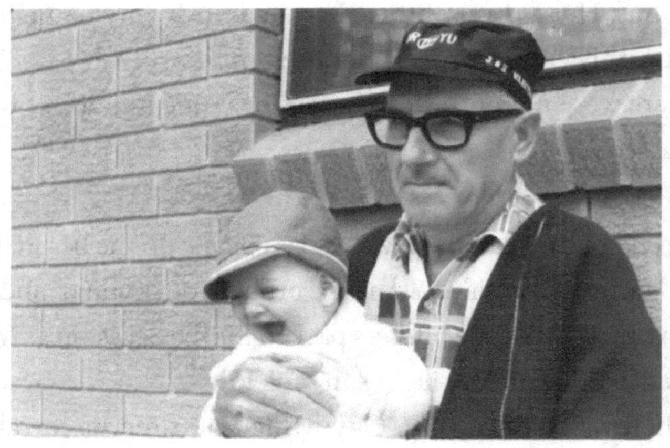

From babyhood, Gerard possessed a capacity for affection that infected others, not the least his previously formal grandparents.

Gerard and his Pa were inseparable. A child on the brink of active and joyful discovery of the world, and a calm, patient man with life and strength diminishing, cherishing every day.

They watched television, sharing the joy of Donald Duck and Bugs Bunny. The house was filled with the piercing notes of toddler hilarity, mixed with the low, manly rumble of my father's laughter.

When Dad was no longer able to put his arm around Gerard, Gerard climbed into his Pa's lap, grabbed his grandfather's arm, pulled it around him and said, 'Come on, Pa, make an effort and help a boy.' Dad's laugh would set Gerard off, and they would giggle hysterically. All Gerard knew—he made his Pa happy. It was enough—enough for both of them.

Gerard coped with his grandfather's decline in the natural way of a trusting child. When his precious Pa died, Gerard grieved deeply. There was no longer the sound of laughter in the house.

A clever bloke

'Good grief, Dad. That looks like a whale skeleton,' I said.

'You've got an imagination there, Bub, I'll give you that.' Dad continued to plane the curved boards with rhythmic precision, clearly enjoying my confusion. 'How's the surface going on that frame, Pete?'

My brother ran a practised hand over the timber. 'Feels pretty smooth, Dad.'

'Good, son.'

There was a load of washing for me to hang on the clothesline, but as usual, Dad's projects held greater appeal than any form of domesticity. 'Can I…?'

'You'd be a help if you tied Snoopy up somewhere else, Sis,' said Peter.

'Aww, leave off! He's too strong for me. He runs round in circles, winding the chain around my legs and pulls me over.' I eyed Snoopy with reluctance, and received his usual tongue lolling grin and thumping tail greeting. 'Anyway, where'll I put him? There's only the clothesline, and I have to hang the washing out.'

Peter rolled his eyes.

Dad looked up and pointed to the back step where Mum stood, hands on her hips. 'Washing won't hang itself, Linda,' she said.

'Doing it, Mum.'

'You're a heck of a long way from the clothesline and basket for someone who's "doing it", Linda,' she said.

I ran to the clothes basket, threw it in the trolley and lowered the line.

'Forget anything, Linda?' asked Mum.

'Aaaah, I don't think so…'

Mum held out the peg basket.

'Oh. Right.'

'You'd forget your head if it wasn't screwed on,' said Mum. 'Leave the men alone.'

This was usually a scenario my brother was only too pleased to join in, but he was either engrossed in helping Dad or having a day off from teasing me.

Mum smiled at "the men" with pride. Not for her the nagging of weary wifedom over half-completed projects strewn across backyards for years. Dad finished what he started. If Mum ever complained he was taking too long at anything, we kids started an uproar, 'Fair go, Mum. You've gotta be kidding!'

We holidayed at Eraring with an assortment of other families. Years earlier, we'd gone on travelling holidays in the little round caravan Dad built, but more recently, we had been renting cabins on Lake Macquarie.

We often spent Sundays at Shingle Splitters, a point that jutted into the saltwater lake, dividing it into a calm haven on one side and a windswept reedy curve on the other. Sometimes the wind turned, its mercurial gusts rampaging both sides, or the calm one - the side that sloped gently into the saltwater lake. Cobalt-green water crimped in midday breezes as it lapped with metronomic lyric on creamy sand. Tall pines extended to the end of the point.

A hilly area where eucalypts, pines and scrub gathered indifferently allowed children a secret domain, where shrieks of 'You're it, tagged ya' echoed over the water.

Then it all changed. The speedboats came with their growling engines, pristine fibreglass perfection, water-thumping speeds, mile-wide wakes, and spitting spray. They heralded a new kind of weekender—water skiers. We moaned that our peace was ruined, our favourite place had "gone to the dogs".

Even Mum paused crossword puzzling in the shade of a tree to squint at the newcomers and mutter, 'Hmmph.'

Dad got an inscrutable glint in his eye. He and Peter took off on trips to the marina in Toronto.

'Crikey, Max,' said Mum, 'you're not looking at those fancy expensive boats, are you? In our dreams.'

However, come summer, as the fruit of Dad and Peter's backyard efforts, we were the proud owners of a sleek speedboat with a gutsy roar and a dashing blue stripe that Dad had meticulously painted. It spewed smoke with the best of them.

So we learned to ski - and by that I mean Peter morphed into James Bond, while I survived as long as the boat went in straight lines, which didn't happen much. There I went - careening off at a perfect tangent to the trajectory of the boat, where I sank in ignominy and had to be pulled aboard spluttering, with my life jacket choking me.

The legacy of patience

To my eternal gratitude, Gerard inherited his grandfather's patience.

"Softly, softly" was one of my father's phrases, one of his maxims. With a wife like Elsie, he needed it often. She would break the keys off in the garage door, and Dad would respond by saying, 'You can't go at things like a bull at a gate, Else'. My mother would then embark upon a lecture that included all inanimate objects under the heading of gross stupidity. I once heard Dad refer to her as cack-handed.

If she plugged the kettle in instead of the toaster and the toaster refused to work, it was 'a stupid thing'. If my father pointed out her mistake in any way that offended her, the lecture would end with the comment, 'If that is all a person can say, a person should be quiet.' A person usually chuckled, further escalating her sense of martyrdom.

Mum must have had a secret ambition to be a market gardener. She tried to train my brother and me to follow her in pursuit of the perfect garden. My brother, however, was not going to be caught dead weeding flowers in her 'stupid garden' and I was a lost cause because I was 'too slow and wouldn't know weeds from flowers.'

In the yard, there were two hoses for the garden, one on each side of the house, as well as an elaborate watering system for the back garden. On one occasion in her usual hurry to get things done, Mum turned the tap on to one of the hoses, and when nothing happened, she spent ages trying to work out why there was no water coming out of the hose. She blustered that she had felt and heard the water in the hose when she had turned it on, so the 'stupid thing must be working.'

Dad was called to the scene and quickly discovered she'd crossed the hoses over. The hose she had turned on was indeed working and had actually been flooding the neighbour's yard for the past half hour, while she had been lamenting its 'stupidity.' Our neighbours were less than impressed with their soggy backyard.

In response, she embarked on the usual monologue, 'I have to do *everything*; if a person would do something to help a person, then a person would have less to do.' Dad made his usual offer to mow over the flower garden so 'a person would have less to do', an idea that was quickly dismissed as being based not only on stupidity, but on thoughtlessness, an even greater insult.

Dad played the piano by ear. He was self-taught, and he never learned to read music. He made and played his own Hawaiian guitar. Gerard could also play by ear, and I see a bit of my father in Bronson when music transports him to another place. Dad only ever played for the family. Mum enjoyed this, proud of his gift for music, and told us, 'Your father can do anything.'

Dad was gentle with Mum and with us.

Nannie

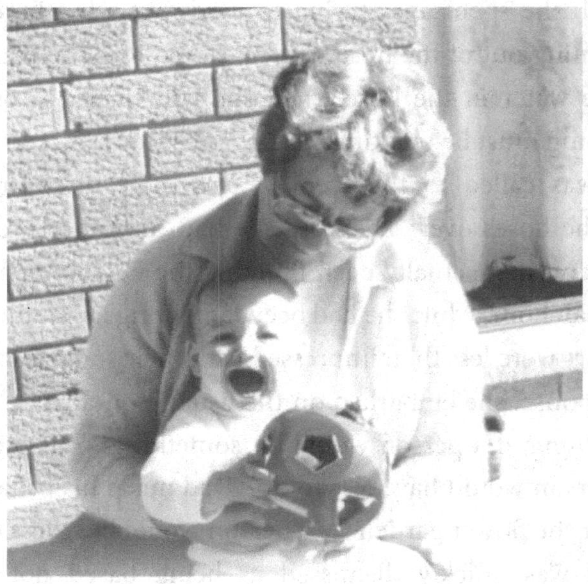

Franz Kafta's *Metamorphosis*, the story of salesman Gregor Samsa who wakes one morning to the shocking reality that he has morphed into a huge insect, details a transformation far less shocking than my mother's transformation from mother to Peter and me to Gerard's "Nannie".

Mum belted my brother and me for crimes and misdemeanours that would've been overlooked in Oliver Twist's poorhouse. She once sent us out to the backyard to source a suitable weapon for punishment. Apparently, we had pushed her patience beyond the pale, and she'd tired of ever making anything of us, the pair of us being hell-bent on remaining heathens.

I chose a thin stick.

'No. NO,' said my brother, clearly more familiar with this torturous system, new to my tender experience. My next choice, a thick plank, was also vetoed.

'Leave it to me, Sis,' he said.

For myself, I didn't see much difference from the precious luggage strap as I screamed blue murder.

"Nannie" would rather take a Valium than lay a hand on a child, certainly not on Gerard, who ruled the kingdom with smiling requests and stern, but gently delivered lectures for her general edification and improvement.

The cherished qualities that made Nannie an immediate and immovable favourite with Gerard did not earn any favour with his mother.

War was declared. Good cop vs better cop. Who won?

The jury's still out.

Before Gerard attended school, he had to attend testing. I had held him back a year, sending him at six, and was roundly chastised for this. After the assessment, I was told that Gerard couldn't read or write his name.

Two weeks later, on Gerard's first day of school, he settled into his desk and gave me an indulgent smile and a wave. I almost expected him to shake my hand and say thanks for the childhood. He sat down with his lunch in the right place, and when he saw that I was a bit teary, he became embarrassed and said, 'It's alright Mum, *you can go now*'. He gave one of the other kids an exasperated look that said 'she can be a bit clingy' and turned to face the front of the class. He was ready to move on.

When I came to pick Gerard up from school several weeks after he started, he was sitting on the opposite side of the classroom from where he began.

'What did he do wrong?' I asked, thinking of my primary school days, where I was shifted all over the place for distracting the others.

'Oh,' said the teacher, somewhat chagrined. 'He is doing Year 2 work, so I moved him over to be with the Year Twos.'

I felt smug because I knew Gerard could read before.

Gerard tolerated school. School tolerated Gerard. Gerard attended school. Although it can be reliably stated that Gerard didn't make his mark there. On the whole, he annoyed teachers, and teachers annoyed him. To alleviate the stultifying discomfort of his formal education, Gerard arrived at that institution as late as he could without drawing unwanted attention.

Nannie took it upon herself to assist Gerard get ready for school, pushing me out of the way as she put Weet-bix in a plate, poured the milk, offered honey, marching back and forth, irritating me enormously. I thought Gerard would be just as annoyed, but he didn't seem to mind her coddling.

On the days that his "helicopter grandmother" was otherwise engaged, Gerard had to get himself off to school. I worked the morning shift (7 am-3:30 pm) at the local nursing home, 5 minutes away.

Mothers are expected to be everywhere. Single mothers are expected to be everywhere, and then some.

Gerard had been late for a week, a fact I discovered by some nefarious means, now forgotten. I realised he was watching telly in the mornings. I gave the usual parental lecture ... 'never again, you hear me'.

Full to the eyebrows of his own importance, along with the accumulated significance of past warlords, conquerors and kings, Gerard boldly said, 'You can't make me.'

In the nurses' staffroom the next day, I sold the telly to whoever would take it far, far away in the lunch hour.

Television gone.

That afternoon, Gerard brought reinforcements to the fray—Nannie sat beside him inside the door in my immediate path when I arrived home. Twin warriors with folded arms and that most tormenting weapon of all, wounded silence.

After a cheery hello, I whistled in the kitchen, feigning the ignorance of The Sublimely Oblivious, knowing my mother had the self-control of a pit bull when a piece of her mind was busting to be shared.

'How dare you,' she said. 'How dare you dispose of the television without consulting that boy.' She pointed at him in case I'd forgotten who he was. "That boy", continued the pained silence saga with the fortitude that comes with childhood, where the only goal in life is to get what they want. After all, bills and life expenses are not present to enlighten or deflect.

'When that boy pays half my mortgage, he'll get a vote,' I said, feeling clever, but doubting that I'd scored any points anywhere but in my own head.

Nanas are not icecream

If Gerard wanted to see Nana and spend time with her, he saw her. She loved him with a tireless, extravagant love.

A love that peeved me to my toes with its constant undermining of my motherhood. But Nanas are not ice cream, treats to be denied, withheld, or measured incrementally.

I challenged her, upbraided, scolded, harangued, reproved.

It didn't change a jot. I dreamed of escape to a quiet, coastal village where the struggling single mother makes a dozen friends overnight and has a handsome neighbour waiting to nurture someone else's child.

Very Mills & Boon and totally bonkers.

She loved him, with a tenacious devotion, as if he were the gift life had denied her, the summation of her dreams. All the affection that she'd been denied, and the affection she'd withheld from her own children, was found in a small boy whose adoration was complete.

When Gerard became a teen, he teased his nana mercilessly and often jumped out from behind doors saying 'boo! 'and this never failed to send her into paroxysms of shock. She never became accustomed to this game, even when she knew he was close by. She reacted as if the worst kind of intruder had invaded her home.

He continued this practice as a young adult and was always amused by her response to the threat of a heart attack and the danger of scaring old ladies.

Once, when she was fully regaled for church with a seemingly double dose of hairspray, he was playing with a cigarette lighter near her, and her hair caught on fire.

Always good in a crisis, Gerard put out the flames with much head-patting, and when she turned her indignation on him, he merely gave her his most angelic smile and told her he had only been patting her because she was a cute nana.

So off she went to church with righteous steps, a scorched and melted patch on her hair, totally ignorant of the antics of the heathens she was leaving at home.

Thankfully, because she had lost her sense of smell she didn't notice the smell of her singed hair.

Gerard had never smoked but always carried a lighter to kill spiders or burn rubbish in the back yard—a practice that sometimes meant the arrival of the local fire brigade.

He would talk his way out of it every time and even have the firemen sit down for a nice chat with a much-diluted warning, and the fire still burning.

Accidental feminist & part-time tyrant

I had skived school and was weighing potatoes in the STAFF ONLY packing and loading area of THE AVONDALE TRADING & CO-OPERATIVE STORE, known colloquially as THE CO-OP.

I made tedious work of this task, choosing potatoes of varying size, putting them on and off the scales, attempting exactness, until Mum asked what the blazes I was doing, then said, 'Just make sure you're over. Always.'

One afternoon, Mum stood at the doorway to the store, eyes narrowed, hands on her hips. After a thoughtful hmmph, that portended trouble, she headed for the front of the store.

'Elsie's on the warpath,' said a shop assistant, grabbing the sleeve of a workmate and pointing at my mother's resolute back.

The prospect of relief from boredom was irresistible, so I followed. Mum's straightforward brutality on matters of work ethics was legendary. She announced her promotion to MANAGER with, 'Let's see how they cope with petticoat government'.

I peeped over the GENERAL CLEANING aisle, pleased Mum had lowered the height of the aisles to survey the activities of 'thieving college students'.

A plump, stylish woman had entered the store and was removing her gloves. She held a nondescript garment wrapped loosely with tissue paper. With head held high, she scanned the store and waited.

'You can't bring that back.' Mum's voice carried over the morning crowd of customers. 'You'll have to pay for it. You've had it too long.'

The woman stalled. It was Mrs Elmore, a formidable dame. A red flush rose from her neck and spread. She turned to face my mother, hands fisted.

The room fell silent with only the chink of the cash register.

'I had this on *appro*[1],' Mrs Ellmore said, 'approved by *you*. I'm returning it.'

'Appro is four days, not "as long as you please"—you've had it for over a month. Most people can ascertain if a garment fits in five minutes, not five weeks.'

The woman stiffened. 'You do know who I am!'

This rhetorical question confused Mum, who lived in a black-and-white world. 'Don't be ridiculous, of course I do.' Mum turned on her heel and walked away.

Mrs Ellmore paused, then smiled and glanced at the onlookers, who developed a sudden interest in the contents of their trolleys.

Early in life, Mum and I had parried over a million subjects. Dad's assessment was that neither of us knew when to leave well enough alone. He was, of course, right. I began as a toddler with questions: 'Why can't my cat talk?' 'Does God wear pyjamas?' 'Who supervises all the money in the world?'

When I was five, I walked into the kitchen while Mum was mopping the floor. This activity involved vigorous swishing that left streaks of water up the wall and was accompanied by loud thumping as the mop hit whatever was in the way, occasionally a

---

[1] "Appro" stands for Approval, a system where customers could take items of clothing home to try on. Garments were taken on trust – there was no payment at the time.

miscellaneous child.

'Get off my clean floor, Linda!' she yelled. 'How many times do I have to tell you blasted kids?'

'But you're on it,' I said, facing certain disaster. 'And your feet are bigger than mine. Why do you walk over the floor while you're mopping it anyway? If you started at the other end, you'd finish in the laundry without walking over it.'

'Look at you, all of five, telling me what to do.' She snorted and gave me The Look— I'd seen her use it on Dad often; the "You're A Right Smart Arse" look.

When I was older, my opinions confounded her as much as my earlier questions. I developed anti-royalist sentiments that she found confronting. She revered the monarchy. We sang *God Save the Queen* at every function, local, church or school. I told her God was not in favour of the monarchical system. I read a text from the Bible where God gave in to the Israelites and let them have a King like the heathens, so they would learn what a ridiculous idea the whole royalty gig was. She was appalled.

The only thing worse than a smart arse was one with God on their side.

Then there's me

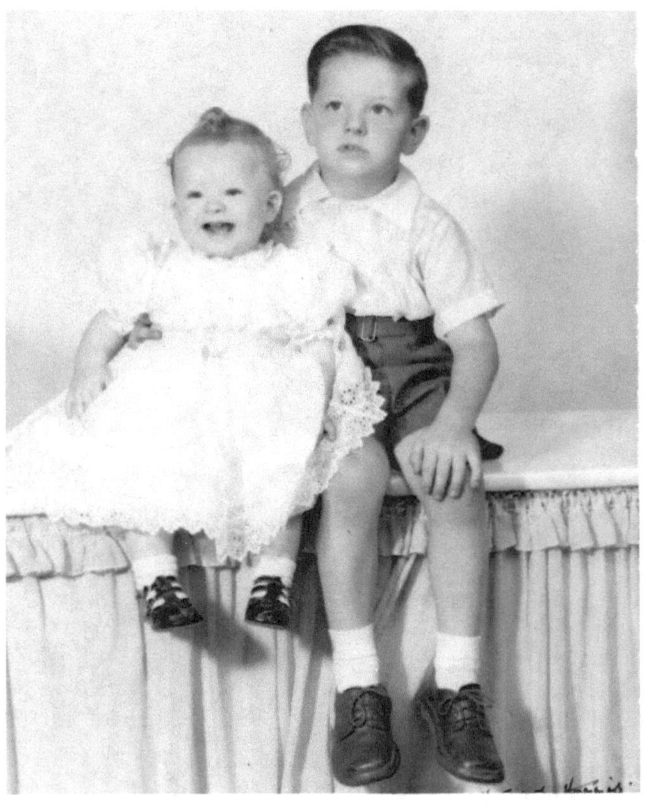

I'm the kid with the curls and the perpetual smile. Mum said I drove her nuts that day because one of my shoes kept falling off. A fair summation of my life, actually.

Early years

Baby

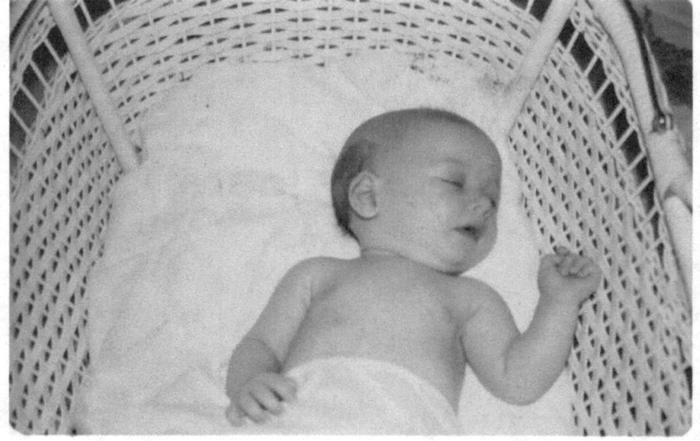

This photo was taken on the day we brought Gerard home from the hospital. Gerard was two weeks old, and I had spent a fortnight in the hospital after a C-section.

Guy had a Christmas "work do" that day and insisted that I attend. I wanted to go home with a newborn, but Guy was adamant. The event was on the way home, so we put Gerard in this basket and set it under the table. Like the hospital staff, people were surprised by his size.

'That's not a newborn. Kid looks 6 months old.'

Gerard was asleep. As is the custom, many people wanted to see the baby.

The noise at the party was boisterous. Gerard slept through the whole thing. The foot-stomping and drunken revery.

When we arrived home, I tried to wake Gerard, fearing he would disturb my sleep later. No matter what I did, Gerard wouldn't wake. Exhausted, I flopped into bed and fell asleep immediately. An hour later, Gerard woke and yowled. He had slept for eight hours. I had slept for one.

However, Gerard only woke for a feed once a night, establishing a routine I could never have instigated. 8 pm feed, six hours sleep, 2 am feed, straight back to sleep, awake and singing at 8 am.

I carried him on my hip, shifting him from one hip to the other. He was heavier than I expected, but I wanted him close. When he wasn't in my arms, he was in a papoose I had made.

Sometimes I just sat, holding him, and singing a mish-mashed lullaby because I could never remember the words.

Sleeping, always a favourite activity, was the only occupation I could achieve for myself without interruption, unlike eating, which caused Gerard to rouse from slumber or play and set up a pitiful wail that would cause evil spirits to flee.

Gerard woke up singing. He sang before he could talk. I shared his afternoon naps. He would stare at me till his eyelids drooped. He would fall asleep with one hand on my face. He was a patter, a comforter, an inscrutable observer. A tender, concerned boy. He would point at his brother's room, say 'bubba', wait for me to put the babe on a pillow on the floor where he would sit, stroking the babe's feet.

His first word was 'Mum', then, seeing my delight, he repeated it.

The next thing he said was a sentence. At eight months of age, he crawled up behind me and said, 'Whatchagot?'

He called himself Douey. Affection was his first language. All anyone had to say to him was 'want one', and he'd pucker up for a kiss.

When Gerard was a toddler, he walked past a candle that was burning too high, and with his bottom lip pursed and his face intense, he thumped the flame out with a chubby baby hand and waddled off with a satisfied air. His instincts were honed and ready early.

That filthy look

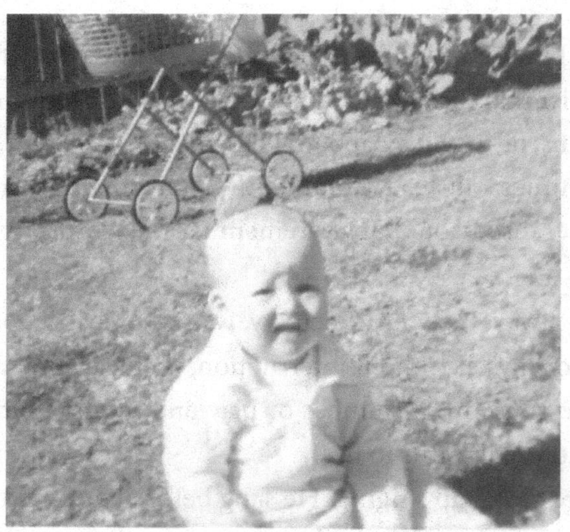

The notorious Infant Filthy Look, established early in life, and used for his often confused parent, and yet not merely restricted to relatives, but brought out to cast disdain on passing randoms.

It was an early sign that "people" per se would not be a favoured species later in life and would only be tolerated in small doses and in even smaller groups.

On this particular occasion, I feel that the placement of a yellow gerbera on his head caused great offence and not a little consternation, but I'm guessing.

It was a look that made its inaugural appearance on the occasion of his first church attendance when his misguided mother put a lace dress on him, one she had diligently repurposed from her wedding gown, a selfless act of great sentimentality and skill.

Not the dummy!

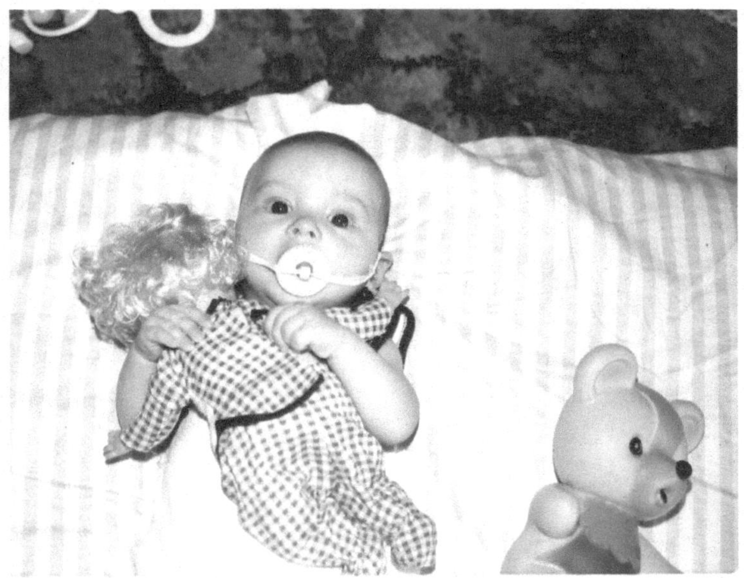

Gerard had an aversion to dummies. He was awake to the honey-dipping trick. I've never seen a kid spit a dummy as quickly and as far as Gerard. They were an insult, fakes designed to fool unsuspecting babes, and he wasn't falling for that.

He didn't cry a lot, so they weren't needed, except during church services where Gerard would mimic the preacher, with gravitas and gusto, grunting and gurgling, in perfect time with the cadence of the pastor's voice, changing the pitch and tone precisely. If the pastor emphasised a point by raising his voice, so did Gerard. 'Har rar rar rar rar har. Hmmph.'

I took the ribbon out of his cardigan and tied his dummy to his ears. It muffled the experience to an acceptable level of audience participation.

I thought this habit was unnoticed until the pastor shook his tiny hand at the door and said, 'Thanks for the help, mate.'

First brother, David:

In spite of using several forms of contraception I fell pregnant again, too soon after Gerard was born.

Guy shared his worry with his family about it. His family expressed their disappointment in me. In their opinion, I should have prevented this from happening. Birth control is a woman's responsibility.

At 28 weeks, I woke to a bed full of blood. On a mad dash to the hospital, Gerard mimicked my moans of labour pain. Our second son was born 12 weeks premature. 3lbs 1oz. There was a lung haemorrhage. The placenta was mince-meat. I was given 3 units of packed cells.

I had been weak and tired, dizzy for weeks before

My preemie underweight baby was wrapped in foil, shown quickly to me, then transferred to a city neonatal hospital. Blood transfusions were also necessary for the tiny boy.

The baby had breathing problems, requiring frequent resuscitation.

When I was finally released from the hospital, I made doll clothes to fit my tiny son. A kind church member delivered my breast milk to my son's hospital.

There were many midnight phone calls.

I needed surgery a month later. There were blood tests for me. Worrying, ominous. Anaemia. Leukaemia? Sternal puncture. Results clear. Slow recovery.

While the little one was still in the hospital, Guy approached me for a talk. He had been speaking with several of the women at church and felt that our baby should be made a ward of the state. There were too many problems. It would be better for everyone.

I shook my head and walked away. I would not give my son away. We didn't even know what effects, if any, would arise from his prematurity.

We brought our new baby home.

Gerard had just begun to walk. His first word in the morning was 'Bubba'. He would drag a pillow from his cot, place it on the ground and say, 'Bubba.'

I would place the little one on the pillow where Gerard would sit beside him and stroke his feet.

Our little preemie died at home six weeks later. He had struggled and failed, fought and lost. And after he died, I was lost. Grief and despair claimed me in equal portions.

One of my dearest school friends sang He Ain't Heavy at the funeral. I was given some money by one of the sweet old ladies at the church to buy a suitable black dress.

I wore white.

It was easier to bear the loss of my baby because I had an armful of wriggling warmth and affection in Gerard. This was compensation. This was comfort.

Guy's boss insisted he take a week off to grieve. He was restless. I wanted to find peace at home in quiet routines and security. I didn't want to haul Gerard here and there, but Guy insisted. He wanted to go somewhere, anywhere. He settled on his paternal grandparents. I loved Grandad Tom and his lovely wife, Phyllis, so I thought it would be okay.

At a hillside cottage where banana plants grew lush and green, we were welcomed with soft, perfumed hugs and crushing granddad embraces. For meals, a table was set with simple fare, salads in crystal dishes, thinly sliced peeled cucumbers and tomatoes. There were crisp, ironed, white sheets. A comfortable place for Gerard, adored by his great-grandparents. A patchwork cotton comforter.

Importantly, there was peace. I was glad we came, until...

On a drifting visit to the Port Macquarie village shops, Guy disappeared, leaving me to comfort Gerard in the stroller on the busy street for hours. I had no money. I had no idea where Guy had gone. Gerard was a patient child, but he began to fret. Guy had the car keys, so I couldn't even wait in the car.

Guy finally returned with a long, slender package. He had been to the local police station and obtained a gun license, then he had been to a gun shop and bought a gun.

I couldn't understand. He had said nothing. A few days after the funeral of our infant son, the thing on Guy's mind was to get a gun.

I was ill at ease. Guy was mercurial on his good days and frightening on his bad days. Why did he want a gun? We lived in a quiet Sydney suburb. He had never gone hunting. He didn't know anyone who went hunting. I fell asleep that night with a rifle under the bed.

In the morning, Guy started packing and said his goodbyes to his grandparents. We were not staying in this peaceful place, but moving on.

A family breaks

First marriage

I have told you some very hard things that nearly broke me with the telling, but I would be remiss if I didn't make some small attempt at describing my first marriage to Gerard's father, Guy, because Gerard was a silent witness to the chaos. It feels a harder subject than many others because he was my first love, the recipient of my innocence and trust, but also the destroyer of those very gifts. It was a tumultuous marriage that lasted four and a half years.

Guy had charisma and knew how to use it. He used it to gain my love and trust, and then it disappeared for me. I saw him use it after that, in church gatherings, with other women and in business, but it would forever be an infrequent visitor to me, and then in hyperbole, overblown rhetoric as the pendulum swung this way, that way. From protestations of undying devotion to cruel obscenities.

I was in *his* life, not he in mine. He knew nothing of my inner life, my hopes and aspirations.

Guy came home from work in the middle of the day for lunch, something he hadn't done before. He ate the meal I had prepared in silence as I hovered nervously. something was hanging heavily in the air. Was it important? He didn't look at me as the fork and knife clattered rhythmically. If it was important, how could he string it out?

He finished the meal, every morsel, set aside his plate and rose. He stood staring out of the kitchen window.

He began to speak in a colourless manner, as if seeking distance from the words, distance from me. The words fell quietly and smoothly, but then began to eddy around the room, taking on a life of their own. He had been having an affair. The midday sun shone through the double doors at the back of the house. The rays slanted to where I stood, brilliantly white. And yet I shivered.

I was wearing a worn dressing gown, a faded, washed-out pink. I remember thinking absently that I should have been looking my best on this most dreadful of days. A wife scorned should look better than an ordinary housefrau.

'Well, do you forgive me?' he asked, his eyes fixed on the clothesline. Anywhere other than on me.

These were his only words, no words of regret, no words of love, sorrow or guilt. His wrongdoing was over. His guilt assuaged. It was now my responsibility. Would we get on with life? Would I forgive, as surely I must?

I could not answer. His question was a careless thing; a waste of words to my wasted heart.

He pressed for an answer.

'Go back to work,' I said. Six months for adultery. Six seconds for forgiveness.

Months later, the car slewed into the driveway at 6 pm. Guy slammed the front door, wrenched his tie loose, and threw his keys on the sideboard. He was in a dark mood. Dark skin, grey-hued, stretched tight across his face. I watched him from the front window of the house where the rubber tree grew wild, threatening the concrete paths. He didn't come back inside for a long time, and when he did, his face terrified me. Was he concocting some punishment for me because I had failed to offer immediate forgiveness for his affair with the schoolgirl?

He brushed past me wordlessly.

Gerard toddled cheerfully down the hall towards his father. I held my breath as Guy put his hand on Gerard's head and steered him aside. Gerard reached for his father, straining toward affection, but Guy walked into the kitchen, where he downed a glass of water, banging it on the sink before leaving the house, heading to the garage. I heard the slam of a cupboard door. The gun cupboard? Oh God.

I saw a shadow as long strides took Guy past the house towards the rubbish tip at the end of the road. It wasn't far. Ours was the last house in the street. I picked Gerard up and ran barefoot up the path. I couldn't see Guy.

A loud bang broke open the stillness.

I felt the air shudder around me, felt it in my blood. Putting Gerard down on the sidewalk, I hushed him, then ran towards the tip, dread threaded along every nerve in my body. Flushed and out of breath, I rounded the bend.

Guy was standing at the edge of the tip, arms folded, waiting.

He smiled, a grim twist of the mouth. 'What's wrong with you!'

A strange night

A fortnight later, arriving home from work late, Guy ignored my greeting. Weaponised silence, a common state. He had not explained his bizarre visit to the tip. He walked around me, as if not seeing me, towering over me, mute to my questions of 'are you okay? What's wrong?' The silence felt as malevolent as the words. As angry as the litany of my faults, abuse for food not being ready early enough, and for the imposition of the needs of a toddler.

Guy had a friend staying over, a teenage boy. Guy spoke soft words to the friend. The air was strained.

I put Gerard to bed. When I came out of Gerard's bedroom, I heard music. Simon and Garfunkel crooned in mellow, mellifluous tones, *I'm a rock, I'm an island.*

Guy was lying in the middle of the lounge room with the rifle, holding it close beside him, barrel up near his face, handle down.

I shook uncontrollably. I was no match for this psychotic morass of twists and turns. My reserves were useless in the path of this tightly-reined internal fury.

Gerard slept in his cot in the back room. Safe. But not safe.

Guy lay splayed like one comatose. I approached, asking, 'What's wrong?' There was no response, not even an eyelash flickered. But Guy was aware, I was sure of it.

The teen was in the kitchen, eyes down, feigning distance from the drama. 'Has he taken drugs?' I asked the boy.

'Er, I...' He turned away.

Soundless and barefoot, I slipped into the laundry. I slid the window open and dropped silently to the path. Navigating dark shadows, I tapped on a neighbour's door, struggling for composure. I made up a story, unsure if I was believed. I phoned our church pastor, a man aware of the chaos. The neighbours' eyes were pained, but how could I tell them of the madness next door? Had they heard my strained words over the phone? 'Come quickly. He has a gun.'

Adrenaline pushed me back through the window.

Car headlights glared into the lounge room where Guy lay with the rifle. Guy leapt up and ran. I watched him take a flying leap over a high timber fence. I insisted that the pastor take the gun. Never to be returned.

I heard the floorboards creak on Guy's return. I feigned sleep in the spare room, fearing to lie beside a greater danger than all the world without.

Guy acted as if nothing had happened in the morning.

I held Gerard close in the morning. Was I protecting him as much as I could? How much of this chaos affected him?

I found a job as the weekend evening supervisor for an aged care village and nursing home. It solved our immediate financial woes.

After only two months, late at night, I stood shivering in a thin jacket on the dark road outside the nursing home, waiting for Guy to pick me up. It was past 1:00 am. It was a thick, dense night. Rain fell. I gathered the jacket around me. I had asked Guy for the car, but he was adamant that he needed it. Where was he? Fear took over. He was not alone. He had Gerard. What was wrong?

Sick of waiting, I returned to the nursing home and phoned Guy's aunt, who lived nearby. I was swiftly retrieved and taken to their home, where I slept indifferently in a strange bed, not knowing where my husband or son could be.

Guy eventually arrived, but without Gerard. 'I left the kid with my brother.'

'He's not even two!' I turned away, angry. Guy's failure to care for Gerard had become a worrying habit.

Guy fumed.

On my next weekend, I arrived home to Guy snoring loudly in front of a snowy, crackling TV. I walked towards him to wake him, but Gerard was screaming, wet and shivering. I bathed and changed him, then took him to the double bed and left Guy sleeping in the lounge room.

Gerard nestled near me. He slept for a few hours, then woke vomiting. He ran to the lounge room, throwing himself on his inert father.

Guy didn't respond. He was slack and unconscious. In red-flagged panic, I assessed him. Ambulance sirens. Quick, efficient ambos. Stomach pumping in the ER. There was no response to my 'I love you. Don't leave me.' I was paralysed by fear, guilt and inadequacy. I was not reason enough. A family with a beautiful son was not enough.

Guy's uncle visited, hugged him and called him an idiot.

I found empty medicine bottles, white dust, broken pills and foil packets strewn over the sink.

I had no way of knowing how long Guy had been like that. How long had Gerard been ill, abandoned?

I could no longer work. Heartsick, I resigned from the job.

Relocation, dislocation

We sold the house and moved, searching for the next Holy Grail solution. With the house sold, we moved back to Avondale, to the seminary. A house was given, free of rent and expenses, courtesy of Guy's uncle, conditional on Guy's continuation with theology.

Guy had bought a brand-new Toyota short-wheelbase 4WD, a crippling financial burden. He often drove to the nearby mountains. One day, he took two-year-old Gerard with him. They were gone for hours. I fretted.

Then down the road they walked, Gerard beside his father.

Guy had tipped the 4WD over. The solution for this was to purchase a winch. I hated driving the thing. Another purchase was a Zodiac inflatable boat. It was great fun on the smooth waters of the creek, but Guy took it into the surf, and every time he did, it overturned, and he had to be rescued.

One morning, while I was gardening, Guy came out of the house carrying Gerard. 'I'm taking the Zodiac out,' he said, slurring.

'No!' I reached for Gerard. Guy increased his grip. The neighbours stared. Guy swore and pushed Gerard into my arms.

Guy brought guests home. A couple from the city church. Unknown to me. 'Stay overnight. Sure, it's fine,' Guy told them.

The bloke was a fancy drug dealer, up from the city to service the students hungry for higher highs or energy for all-nighters. He didn't stay, but his girlfriend did. His business completed, the bloke left, full-pursed. The woman was a full-show cleavage, curvy, troubled addict.

Guy said he was staying up until the early hours with the curvy woman, pushing aside my pleading. To respect me.

All the trust I had pieced together came crashing down. The woman looked like the girl Guy had cheated with, the shape, the curves, the troubled eyes that slanted away from me and fixed on Guy.

With my heart tearing like old satin garments, I fled the house and ran to the nearby cemetery. I lay on our baby's grave for hours, sobbing deeper than the sodden earth beneath me. But when I rose from that damp place, I vowed I would never fall so low again.

Gerard suffered dreadful night terrors. I didn't know what they were at first. Screaming loudly, but not really awake, Gerard was inconsolable. Guy was furious, yelling abuse about the noise and lost sleep. He would never survive with that hullabaloo.

Gerard screamed about cars coming and other strange images. When he screamed, I took him outside to avoid Guy's wrath, then, realising that these were no ordinary sleep disturbances, I took Gerard to my doctor, who prescribed medication that helped him sleep peacefully again.

My doctor was forming a picture of my marriage. When Guy left a cryptic, suicidal message on an exam paper and then disappeared, this doctor was part of the search party.

I left several months later.

After the divorce

After leaving Guy, I lived with my parents and nursed Dad, who
suffered from Motor Neurone Disease.

As I write the stories of Gerard's life, I feel as though I am intruding into the narrative. Gerard was in and around so many events that I will never know the depth of his feelings. In the last three years of his life, he opened up about many experiences and was able to articulate how he had felt, and those conversations were a gift.

How often do we adults converse and come and go, without realising the effects of situations on our children? What did Gerard see? What did he feel? What did he know? A quiet, uncomplaining child, he hardly ever volunteered his perceptions, but would sometimes confide over a chocolate milkshake and hot chips. A ruse I was happy to use to help him open up. Sometimes it worked, sometimes it didn't. However, when it came to my mother and father, and Gerard's Uncle Gordon, there was never a doubt. He loved and trusted them with a fierce devotion that shaped the man, husband and father he became. And the son with whom I was privileged to rattle along life's highway.

Gerard was there in late January when a sultry breeze eased the heat of a summer's day that was perfect for outdoor fun. I set up a wading pool in the front yard of my parents' home.

It was Guy's scheduled weekend for access, but he hadn't been turning up half the time, leaving Gerard staring at the door with his small suitcase beside him. A patient child, Gerard, often sat for over an hour waiting. With this uncertainty and Gerard's disappointment, I decided to pack his things and put them aside, only telling him about access when his father arrived, if he arrived.

Soon Gerard's friends were revelling in the cool water and playing with water pistols. The time for Guy's arrival passed. He was an hour late. I threw on a swimsuit, fetched a garden hose and joined the fun with the kids.

Guy arrived, slewing gravel.

Uninvited, he came inside when I went to collect Gerard's backpack.

'Why are you in the front of the house dressed like that?' Guy said, 'Don't you ever think how I might feel? You're still my wife.'

I ignored his remarks and handed him the suitcase.

'You will never find another man to love you as I do, Linda.'

'I'm counting on it,' I said.

Guy called Gerard to come, but Gerard hesitated. He had become more reluctant to go with his father. When I asked him why, he said, 'Dad only does stuff he likes. Not nice things for a kid. Dad makes me sit in a speedboat for ages. It's very bumpy.'

'Come on, Gerard. Time to go,' said Guy.

'I haven't finished playing with my friends, Dad.'

Guy turned to me. 'You're turning the kid against me. I see what you're doing.'

'You don't think it's related to you at all? Not turning up. Doing your own thing when he's with you?'

Gerard was there when Guy ran to the side storeroom of the house and grabbed several paintings, artwork that was part of the divorce settlement. Galloping to the car, he sped off.

Inside the house, I saw thick tears rolling down my father's cheeks. 'Oh Dad, are you alright?'

Dad shook his head, unable to speak. Dad first noticed a weakening of muscle strength in his right arm, and then he was diagnosed with Upper Motor Neurone Disease.

The disease was progressing, and with it, Dad's sense of helplessness increased. His speech and swallowing were becoming affected.

'Tell Guy that he is not to come inside anymore, Linda,' my mother said, 'he has no respect for us. Not any more.'

Mum put her hand on Dad's shoulder. 'To think of all we've done for him and he can't show even the smallest sign of human kindness to us. I paid his school fees. We put him through high school.' Mum stiffened. 'I bought everything he needed, down to his underwear. I will tell him if you don't.'

For the first time, I realised how deeply Mum had been hurt, for herself and for Dad.

It distressed Dad that his movements were slow, that he didn't have time to stand and walk to the door to have some semblance of protective manhood during Guy's visits, on the next occasion…

Gerard was there after Dad organised his brother-in-law's presence for the next access visit. Gordon was Mum's big brother, a man who had served as a stretcher-bearer in the Second World War.

Uncle Gordon only had to make a brief appearance to severely impinge on Guy's ability to converse and threaten.

Gerard was there, a week later, when Dad came out of the shed balancing a four-pronged walking aid and a bag of tools.

'What are you doing, Dad?' I asked.

'You'll see, Bub.'

Two uncles arrived to assist with the new project.

After a weekend away, I found that the outdoor storeroom had been transformed. It not only had an impressive-looking deadlock, but it was now a kitchenette.

Dad proudly announced that there were two rooms that were my new living space. One room for Gerard and a bed-sit/kitchen for both of us.

My parents' house no longer felt like a temporary respite, but a place of my own.

Guy could no longer intrude.

Gerard was there when I learned to cut fibro and mix plaster.

Hammer in hand, I was often at the top of some table or chair, taking instructions from Dad.

We tackled the hole where Guy put his foot through the ceiling when he was drunk.

After filling the hole with chicken wire, I scrunched up newspaper and shoved it into the chicken wire. Then Dad showed me how to mix spackle to the right consistency. We used buckets of the stuff to fill that hole.

We celebrated the finished job with a block of Dairy Milk chocolate.

This was a rare treat because Dad had trouble swallowing chocolate. I teased him that he would have to drink a bucket of milk to help get it down.

'It's worth it,' he said.

Gerard was there when Guy brought him back early from access. Guy was fiddling with something on the front seat of the 4WD as I walked over to him to collect Gerard's backpack. Guy stood, anger etched on his face. I stalled.

Guy opened the door of the car, watching me with a grey, stony face. There was a newspaper on the front seat with a full colour spread. An incident on the outskirts of a nearby town.

FOUR DEAD IN FAMILY HOMICIDE

An estranged husband threw a firebomb into a caravan belonging to his in-laws, killing his ex-wife, her parents and their child.

Guy smirked. 'You could be on the front page of the paper too.'

Cuddle my feet, Mum

Somehow I have to tell you this
now when you're only three
to try to get across to you
how much you mean to me.

Because maybe one day
you'll stand in front of me
with fire in your eyes
and I will know for myself
that sinking feeling
only a parent knows
that you've lost something.

So now,
while your tiny chubby hand
is reaching down
from the top bunk
to hold mine,
I will listen to you say,—

'My word, those plants are growing.
Cuddle my feet, mum.'

*Written when Gerard was three.

Kidnapped

The phone rang at the nursing home where I worked every second weekend. It was Mum. 'Linda! Linda! I don't know what to do. Guy hasn't brought Gerard back. He was supposed to be here by 2 pm, and it's 4 pm. He hasn't phoned or… He's had an extra two days. The holiday traffic isn't that bad. What can we do?'

A friend set me up with her boss, a solicitor. An ex parte court order was necessary. Frank was vigilant and thorough in obtaining this, an arduous process.

I assumed Guy would be with his older brother, so I called there and asked for him. Guy's brother was shocked. 'How did you get my number? I mean …' his nervousness alerted me.

'I know Guy is there with you. Police are involved. I have a court order and …'

'He'll be leaving soon.' An urgent tone.

I wasn't far away, not the hours they assumed. I had phoned from a payphone up the road.

'Guy wants to say something,' said the brother.

Guy took the phone, 'I'm not bringing Gerard back. He's my son.'

There was a click of the phone.

Less than an hour later, at the police station near the turf farm, a tall officer attended to me. I related my story, telling the officer that Guy often didn't turn up for access and had refused to bring Gerard home.

The officer said, 'Ah, deadbeat dads, waste so much of our time. Control freaks usually. The court phoned us, love. We've phoned the farm, turf isn't it? And we've been out there. The kid's alright. Some family is there. Got a mouthful from your ex. Contradicted himself.'

'Oh. I didn't realise you had a warning.'

'Yep,' said the officer. He tapped a large, flat book on the desk. He opened it and winked. 'Can you read upside down?'

I nodded.

'I'll get you a cuppa and get another officer to go out there.'

I read, shocked by Guy's lies. He claimed to have my blessing and that I was making trouble.

When the officer returned, he said, 'We know. Bunch of lies, love. The idiot doesn't know that we have copies of the court documents sent to us.' He shook his head.

'However, there is some bad news, pet. We don't actually have the power to enforce the return of your son. It will rely on you to convince your ex. Sorry about that, but it's the law.'

'Oh dear, I've never been able to convince Guy to take out the trash. What hope have I got?' I muttered.

'Don't undersell yourself, love. It has taken spunk to drive here and talk calmly. You'll do fine.' He led me to the police car where another officer was waiting.

In the car, the officers chatted freely to me about Guy's demeanour.

'Arrogant twit. Acted like the Lord of the Manor. We see lots of idiots like that, more bluster than substance.'

It was an isolated rural area with no neighbouring properties.

When Guy saw me with the two police officers, he spoke politely and ushered us inside. Ironically, he was wearing a pair of pyjamas I sewed for him.

The senior policeman spoke. There was a tedious back-and-forth with Guy giving no ground. Gerard was playing with toys on the floor. He said, 'Daddy has fireworks, and I want to see them.'

I stepped into the conversation. There was a noticeable change in Guy. He flushed and stiffened his stance, then gestured grandly to his wide-eyed guests and said, 'Look what I have to put up with. See!'

'Yes,' I said, 'they see. I have the courage to act openly. Unlike your treatment of me, carried out behind closed doors.'

Open-mouthed, Guy slumped onto a nearby low lounge, with no further words to offer.

I gathered Gerard, his suitcase and toys, and left, with the police officers following.

Gerard was thrilled to be in a police car and sit in the front on one of the officers' laps. 'Can you put the siren on?' he asked.

The officers laughed. 'Wait a bit, sonny, we'll put it on down the road a bit. Don't want to upset the applecart.'

Down the road a bit, the siren blared.

Sanctuary

After Guy's threats and his failure to return Gerard, my solicitor advised me to find sanctuary somewhere until the final custody case, somewhere Guy wouldn't find her.

I was handed a train ticket and a name—Eva.

We would be met at the train. Gerard, then three, carried an air of delight, thrilled with the prospect of travel. He asked no questions of where or why. 'Oh, good, Mum. We will have an adventure. I like adventures.'

As soon as we were on the train, I sighed with a new kind of relief, unexpected and welcome. My throat was so tight I had trouble speaking. Gerard, always intuitive of my distress, saw my relief and became engrossed in the passing scenery. All around, other children harried their weary mothers, but Gerard revelled in the tranquillity of being near a mother free from anxiety, a state he was too familiar with. How I hated that my shroud of pain affected my son.

The station was tiny and open-air, more of a siding, perhaps only the length of two carriages. Gerard manfully struggled with his small colourful suitcase, refusing help as we gathered our belongings. My fears of not finding our hostess were washed away when I saw only one person on the platform, a woman holding a straw hat firmly on her head, scanning the train, her floral dress billowing gently in the breeze. I knew she was waiting for us. I walked into Eva's embrace, her soft, generous body comforting me.

'You're here now,' was all Eva said, picking up the suitcase as if it were a feather. She led us to a little blue Corolla and chatted brightly, as if we were old friends continuing a conversation begun the day before. Eva told me she and her sister, Lil, had spoken with the local police officer, reassuring me that I was safe.

Eva went about her days as if we had always been there, seamlessly including us.

We strolled through country lanes. Eva talked nonstop, while Gerard dragged a stick in the dusty trails, and my mind wandered to yesterday's fears and tomorrow's battles.

Eva's house was a lone house in a picturesque valley where the road wound upward, and a creek bubbled through and beyond, pure water over polished stones.

Gerard and I grew carefree and relaxed, wandering the gentle hills, the lush valley. We were miles from anywhere, in a world of stillness and green, so much green. All our stories and conversations began with "we two". We sang 'You and Me Against the World' as we lay by the pebbly creek, Gerard's head resting on my stomach.

'You have a sweet voice, Mummy,' Gerard said, beginning to hum.

Tears pricked my eyes. We threw pebbles against the rocky bank of the small creek, squealing with glee when the stones bounced back to us, the sound echoing through the lush valley.

'We're very distant, aren't we, Mummy?' said Gerard. His language was not like that of his small friends. There was a quirky, profound quality to his speech that amused and confused his friends and delighted the adults he met. Some older boys, Eva's nephews, came to visit. One of the boys said to Gerard, 'Don't go into the kitchen, there's jelly all over the floor.'

'Don't be ridiculous,' said Gerard.

The two boys giggled at three-year-old Gerard.

Eva's sister Lil lived nearby. I stayed with Lil and her husband Joe, higher in the mountains, for a few days while Eva visited a sick friend. Lil was a large woman with a hearty laugh and a ready smile. Gerard and I slept in bunk beds with a view of the valley. I helped out in the kitchen where a huge timber table dominated the room, and a wood-fire stove radiated warmth.

'Think you're up for a bit of wood chopping, Linda?' asked Lil.

'Sure, Lil, I often chopped kindling and small logs as a kid.'

I managed to get the axe stuck on my second strike at the thick, round log. Embarrassed beyond belief, I tried every trick in the book to free the axe. I thumped it with other blocks of wood, then tried to gain leverage with my weight. I failed to move the damned axe a millimetre. Humbled, sweaty and defeated, I confessed to Lil.

'I saw you from the window.' Lil gave a hearty, full-throated roar of laughter. 'Well, that's no surprise. There's nothin' of you.'

Lil went out to free the axe, and I followed.

'What kind of blasted wood is it anyway?' I muttered darkly.

This sent Lil into another peal of laughter. 'Well, it's good to see some spirit in you, girl.'

In one effortless swing after another, Lil demolished the entire wood pile as if it were butter. I watched in awe and carried the cut timber inside to the basket beside the open fireplace.

Gerard and I joined Lil's husband Joe as he herded his small herd of cattle to another paddock. Gerard ran along with Joe, yelling 'Yar, Yar,' and waving a stick like Joe.

Lil asked me to collect eggs from the chooks. There was a large, enclosed run. 'Watch out for the rooster,' she said. 'He's a screecher. Doesn't like strangers. Got those sharp spurs. Watch out for them. You'll be right.'

I took the bucket and entered the pen, and was immediately set upon by a fierce rooster that took menacing hopping strides towards me, wings out. Terrified, I ran out.

Gerard calmly took the bucket, went inside, wandered through the long, convoluted run, collecting eggs here and there as he went. Not once did the blasted rooster make a sound or fly at Gerard.

'What's the matter with you, Mum?'

When Gerard was eight, I bought a house up the road from Mum and Dad. There was a chook pen, so I got some laying hens. Gerard loved them. He hatched some chickens in his bedroom with a light, cotton wool and a shoebox.

I went outside one day, and all I could see were white bundles of feathers. I panicked and called Gerard.

Gerard came out and said, 'Oh, that. Don't worry. I hypnotised them all.' He then picked one up and demonstrated his new skill.

We eventually got two Rhode Island Red roosters, but that's another story.

Threats

A friend approached me and asked if I wanted to job-share a medical collection job, picking up pathology samples from various medical centres and delivering to a pathology centre. The good news was that the hours were good, and it came with a car. The bad news was that the car was a Leyland P76 that might jolt to the wrong side of the road if it hit as much as a pebble.

On the first day, I took Gerard with me. It was after an access weekend. Gerard slept for the whole five-hour trip. He told me, 'Daddy gave me a little yellow tablet.'

At the family court, in the ladies' toilets, women chain-smoked and swallowed Valium to calm their nerves.

Guy sat closely beside me in the waiting area. He sat arms folded until he got annoyed with my indifference, stormed out of the room and rang a former girlfriend, loudly enough for the whole place to hear. He left the room, returned, ranted and raved, and came back periodically to add another threat. He would take this from me in court. He would take that.

Days before the hearing, he said, 'If you reject me, I will reject our son. If I can't be father, I won't play uncle'.

It was a promise he kept.

Guy moved to America when Gerard was five. Guy requested a goodbye lunch with Gerard and me. Mum and Dad waited in the car in the car park.

Guy spent the whole time trying to talk to me about going back to him, even though we had been divorced for over two years.

Gerard got up, left and went to the car. 'Dad wasn't interested in me. He just wanted to talk to you,' he said.

And yet, Gerard grieved. For the rest of his life, there would be a hole in his heart that only his father could fill.

Laughter and love

For those early years after the divorce, Gerard and I were two pals going to the beach together, building sand sculptures, eating pizza and ice-cream, and riding on the dodgems.

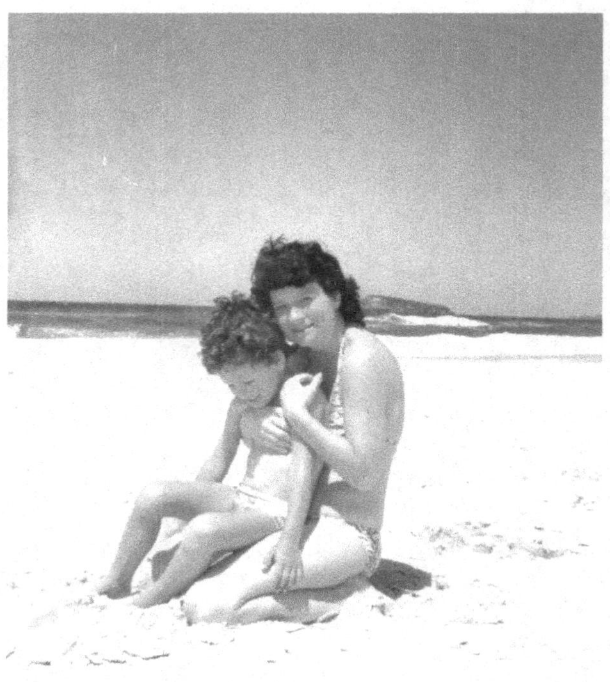

The script

Every family has a script. The family that says they have no script merely means they have the Anything Goes script. In some families, gatherings are calm affairs without tension or disagreement. Great effort is made to ensure the conversation flows with ease, and good manners are maintained. It is an unspoken rule that family issues are buried and ignored. Other families have a riotous script where everyone voices their opinions and feelings, either having a wonderful time or leaving emotional debris in their wake.

In every family, the script flows seamlessly until a newcomer arrives and upsets the applecart, someone unaware of the unspoken rules that dictate the family rhythm.

I was once visiting a friend whose husband was narrow and inflexible, rigid and rule-bound. I inadvertently stepped into the finely tuned balance of their family script.

Gerard was about five, and he was playing with their daughter, Emma, who was the same age.

I was out in the yard with the children, watching them play and chatting. Emma was telling Gerard in an authoritative voice that there was a tiger in the tree, and Gerard was happily responding by saying it was very silly; there was no tiger in the tree, but there was a hippopotamus in the wading pool.

I entered the conversation with a monkey or two of my own when my friend's husband came upon this nonsense. Picking Emma up by the arm, he intoned, 'Don't tell lies, Emma, there is no tiger in the tree, *is there?*' he said sternly.

'Yes, there is, Daddy.'

Whack.

'Don't lie! There is *no* tiger in the tree, *is there?*'

'No, daddy.'

Gerard and I were left standing outside, pondering our sanity, as the man went inside, taking his imaginative daughter, with the satisfied air of having set the world to rights about the matter of non-existent zoos in his front yard.

Gerard quietly slid his hand into mine and gripped it tightly. 'There *is* a hippopotamus in the pool, isn't there, Mummy?'

I replied that I was sure there were actually several.

This man didn't discern the difference between childlike imagination and a lie. I was also sad for the child who was forced to see the world through this narrow, distorted lens and who believed she had done something wrong.

Health struggles

When Gerard had surgery at three years of age, I slept beside him on a thin mattress on the floor, and when the nurses complained that I was in the way, I put the mattress under the bed and slept there instead.

Gerard was in a six-bed, and he never whimpered, but would pat my arm and say, 'It's OK, mummy'.

He slept like a dream at night and never woke, and needed me. Or perhaps he slept because he knew I was there.

This was not true for the other five children in the small ward. One had had a tonsillectomy and vomited on and off throughout the night. He was too sick and too young to ring for help, so I held his head while he threw up and rang for the nurses. The other children were suffering from various illnesses, and all through the long nights, I would be up ringing the bell for them and generally making a nuisance of myself. I did not get the impression that the staff appreciated my ministrations. The number of times that they told me that there were armchairs in the waiting room down the hall told me this.

When Gerard was eight, he developed severe psoriasis. He had huge patches on his elbows and knees, over his back and through his hair.

He was teased relentlessly at school.

He didn't scratch it through the day, something I would never have managed, but at night, in his sleep, he scratched at his head until it bled. I tried cortisone creams with some benefit. I put it through his hair at night with a plastic cap.

We tried everything, warm oat baths…

It was related to stress, so I tried to keep things calm. I didn't insist he attend school swimming events.

One day, he came to me and said he was not going to have steroid creams anymore. I asked him why, and he said he had watched a documentary about cortisone and the side effects.

I hadn't heard about this, and couldn't remember watching a documentary with him, but Gerard often chose to watch documentaries rather than cartoons.

We tried alternative therapies after that. Therapies that Gerard had researched and accepted.

I was never the boss with Gerard. He was quiet and sensitive. I was haunted by his father's suicide attempts and the glimpses into the tortured soul of his father that profoundly affected me throughout that marriage.

I gave Gerard soft love, afraid to break him, as I had seen his father broken. I would always see Guy's eyes in the eyes of my firstborn son. I had been helpless in the wake of the currents and undercurrents of his father's anguish.

However, along with his sweet nature, Gerard had a quiet, determined will of iron. He could go the distance and then some. He outmanoeuvred me every step of the way. The words 'immovable object' come to mind. I spent my mothering days with him, trying to get him to start, and my days with his brother getting him to stop.

I think one of the biggest crocks offered as parenting advice is the 'treat every child the same' philosophy. The concept of a child's individual currency made more sense and was more successful.

For some children, a time-out works.

If I sent Gerard to his room for time-out, he simply climbed onto the bed and went to sleep. Time out worked for him; he loved it! It was, however, a disaster at making any kind of point.

That's what best friends do

'I have to go to a funeral, Mum.' Gerard approached me in the kitchen, with a calm, serious face. Manly demeanour. Nine years old.

'Oh,' I said. With any other child I would have started a discussion.

'Mum. You can drop me off. It's on Tuesday. Next week. Michael's sister. She died of a weird kind of cancer. Something in her abdomen. Really rare.'

'Yes, a horrible loss for them. That's a wonderful thing. For you to do.'

'I didn't know her, but Michael is my best friend. And that's what best friends do for each other. I'm going for him.'

I was too choked up to answer.

'I don't want to be late, Mum. I don't want to ride my bike there. I want to be dressed up properly and not mess up my clothes riding my bike. But, Mum. I don't want to be late. I don't like being late. You are sometimes late, so…'

'I won't be late. I promise.'

'Thank you. I appreciate it.'

'Is it okay if I stay, don't just drop you off?' I asked.

'If you want to. I know you like the family, and Michael. The Hansen's are great people. Mrs Hansen was my best pre-school teacher and she makes great peanut butter sandwiches. And Mr Hansen, well, he's really funny. I love visiting their house. I guess it will be okay if you want to stay for the funeral. I'm fine to go alone. You won't cry a lot will you?'

'No. I'll be okay.'

Gerard stood solemnly amid the mourners, listening intently to the service, head bowed for prayer. Standing tall. Quiet and resolute. It wasn't important that I was beside him as he looked straight ahead, still and calm.

He sang the hymn with reverence.

He left my side. He was the only child to join the queue to give his condolences to the mourners. Dr Hansen, his wife, Michael, Michael's grandmother. He shook hands with them all, murmuring soft words that I could not see. He handed Michael's mother the card he bought and wrote in. I didn't even know he had it.

He didn't notice the stares from the other mourners. Curiosity for a child more like a man. Waiting patiently, he didn't omit anyone from the family, whether he knew them or not. He didn't care if he was watched and commented on.

Gerard would not walk in front of a crowd to accept a first prize ribbon after winning a running race, but he didn't think twice of being noticed, honoring his friend.

After the service was over, Gerard turned to me, as if remembering I was there too, he said, 'We can go now, Mum.'

Gerard jettisoned his Sunday best when we got home. He didn't like getting dressed up and only wore conservative clothes.

He never wanted bright colours or Brand name clothes.

I often felt bad that I couldn't afford to buy him the latest fashion so he would be like his friends, never realizing that he hated any clothing that drew attention to him. I used to go to Op Shops and take the fashion labels off, and stitch them to his clothes, his baseball hat, his hoodies. I sewed T-shirts and hoodies in fashionable styles.

It made me feel better. He had the same kind of clothes as his friends.

It had the opposite effect on Gerard. 'Please stop doing that, Mum. I don't have to dress like my friends. I don't like those fancy things.'

He was like that all his life, choosing traditional clothes while I longed for fashion and style for myself.

Over the years I bought him track pants and hoodies for birthdays and Christmases, always remembering the narrow range of his likes and dislikes.

When he returned to stay with me after the divorce, I was shocked when bought a colourful hippy jacket.

I took a while for me to face distributing his clothes after he died. People suggested numerous ways to remake the jacket, a cushion., etc… Sell it, give it away.

But I couldn't part with that hippy jacket. I couldn't remake it. I won't remake it. It is fine as it is. No renovation needed. For the jacket, or the son.

Chooks, roosters & a mad dog

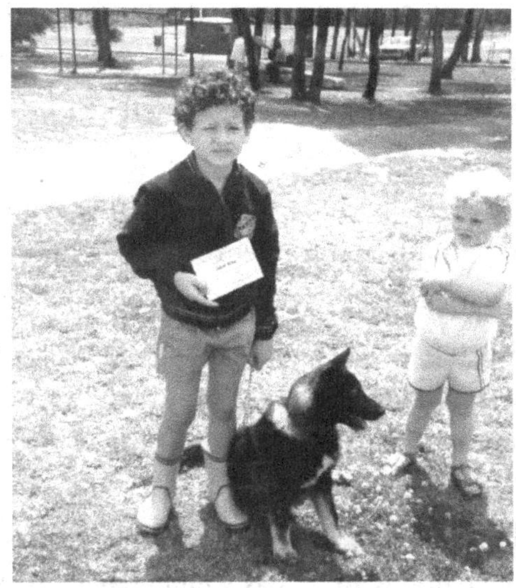

I purchased a home I loved for Gerard and me, just down the road from Mum and Dad, in the street where I grew up.

I once knew a boy named Tristan. He was the four-year-old son of a big, square, competent guy whom I dated between marriages. He was the kind of boy the writer of 'Ginger Meggs' had in mind. With wispy fine blonde hair curling out at all angles, he looked like a wild angel. His beguiling blue eyes were huge and constantly overflowing with surprise. He was a traffic stopper. *Literally.* If horns blared in the street, you could bet a King's ransom that Tristan was in the street, stopping traffic. His father had his own unique style of reality therapy for this kind of behaviour. After said incident, he would take Tristan out the back of the house and tell him in the strongest terms that his life would be cut short, he would never live to play with his toys again. He would be dead and buried in a hole with the dirt "banged on top". The boy's eyes would grow as large as saucers. All would be well until the fire brigade came down the street. A good five minutes later. Horns blared. Back to the drawing board. Or in this case, the backyard to demonstrate a hole with the dirt banged on top. The frequency of this behaviour smacked strongly of the point not being taken.

Gerard was eight at the time and had a dog named Monty. This erratic, loveable mutt, a cross between a German Shepherd and a Husky, had been named by his previous owners because of his love for Monte Carlo biscuits. The dog's frenetic curling tail was at comical variance to his dark, intense face. We strongly suspected that Monty had been given marijuana, which was a part of the previous owner's staple 'diet'.

Tristan also had a dog, or more correctly, his father did. Cindy was an ex-police dog who was as well behaved as the boy was not. She seemed to experience great embarrassment on finding herself in the many precarious situations Tristan placed her. Her eyebrows twitched, and her noble face was awash with apology. She would stand obediently at attention while Tristan lifted her tail and tried to insert a stick. After the disciplined life of a police dog, it must have been extremely trying to find herself with a four-year-old who would have given Attila the Hun a run for his money.

One day, Tristan decided he would talk to the rabbit that was on loan from the school. It was Gerard's privilege to have the class pet for a weekend. Soon, the cry went out from the neighbours that the rabbit was on the loose. Cindy lay down and cried. Monty took chase and cornered the rabbit three doors down, with Gerard in hot pursuit and the rest of us following. Monty, who had eaten all of our chicks soon after they hatched, seemed, for some reason, strangely reluctant to sink his teeth into the rabbit. The rabbit was rescued and returned to its hutch, its heart racing. On questioning Tristan, he said, 'I didn't leck the rabbit out, it lecked itself out.'

Not content with this feat, Tristan decided to follow this gag up by putting both dogs in the chicken coop that housed Gerard's adult hens and two grossly proud Rhode Island Red roosters. Cindy retreated to the corner of the coop and put her paws over her eyes. Monty pursued the colourful roosters round the enclosure, and by the time we arrived, they were missing their tail feathers and much of their pride. Both roosters refused to come out of the coop until their feathers had regrown. Tristan was punished by having to lie on a bed for half an hour's time out. During this time, he managed to sneak into the kitchen and polish off an entire packet of Kingston creams. However, he was unable to blame anyone else, as he was covered in biscuit crumbs.

Tristan had two very sweet Nanas. Tristan didn't swear. He made up for this character defect by telling people to 'ping off'. He once tried this neat trick on Gerard's stocky, no-nonsense Nan, my mother. Wrong move. Little Red Riding Hood would have been relieved to find the wolf in this granny's bed. You get the picture. There was no quiet lecture on manners. That day, Tristan got the true meaning of what it was to 'ping off'.

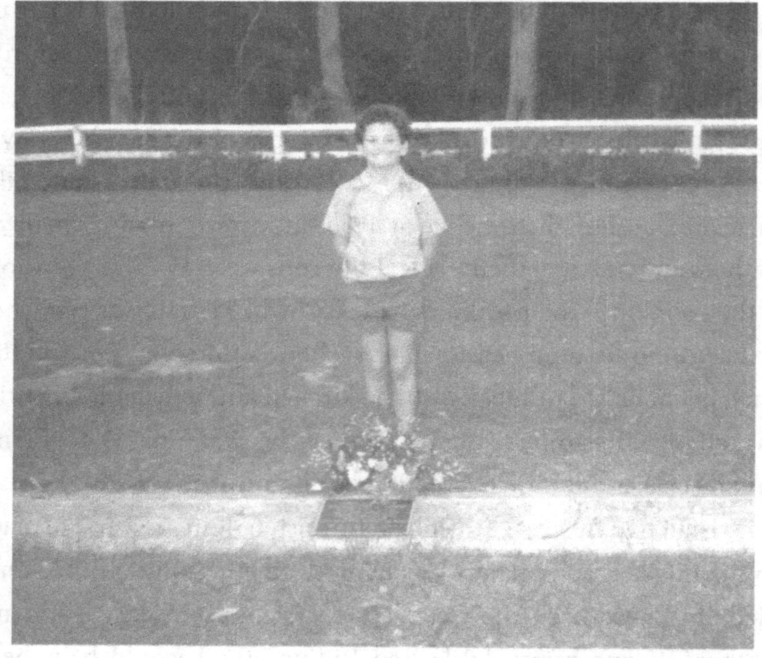

A loss

Gerard mourned his Pa. He stood like a sentinel for this photograph at the cemetery near the grave of his beloved grandfather.

My workplaces

When Gerard was five, I took him to the nursing home where I worked to acclimatise him for the time when his beloved grandfather would need nursing home care. I never wanted Gerard to shrink at the sight of his Pa. He sometimes spent time there when I was on duty.

The nursing home was owned and run by an Italian family, and their children had the run of the place. Children of staff members were always welcome in the nursing home or at the nearby family home, giving them a natural view of the elderly and disabled.

Gerard would wander around unseen and unheard, helping, even though I told him that it was all right to just sit in the TV room with the patients. If there was a tussle over food in the dining room, he quietly and calmly removed the food and told the patients he would only give it back when they stopped fighting over it. They accepted his authority. He often sat and fed someone while he watched cartoons.

We had a woman named Molly who was particularly aggressive in the evening. She fought like a tiger and screamed like a banshee after tea. Out would come the sedative injection, and then it would be a slow tussle all the way to bed.

One night, I couldn't find Molly. There wasn't the usual commotion in the corridors.

Gerard approached me and said, 'If you're looking for Molly, I told her she looked tired and needed to go to bed.'

Sure enough, there was Molly asleep in her own bed.

One afternoon, Gerard interrupted me while I was receiving the handover report from the previous RN, minutes after our arrival. He pointed and said, 'Excuse me, Mum, that man in there is dead.'

When I asked if he wanted to be a nurse, Gerard said, 'Get real, Mum! That is the last job on earth I'd want to do.'

Later, when he was eight, Gerard came to the preschool where I worked. While there, he loved taking one of the little tots up and down the slide.

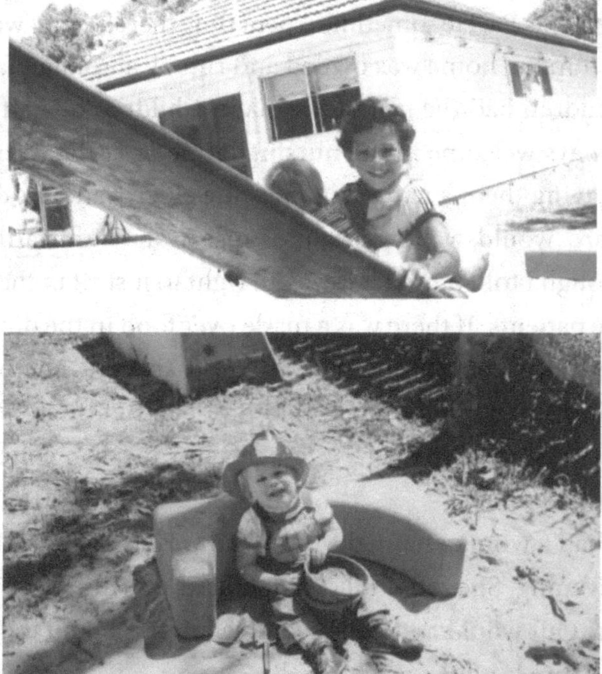

Gerard would sit and play with Duncan, a boy with cerebral palsy.

School excursion

I lined up with the other parents, wondering if any of them were as anxious as I was to assist the teachers on a primary school excursion. An excursion to a place that I hated visiting, The Reptile Park at Gosford.

Gerard was eight and well-behaved, so I thought I would have a nice wander around the park with him, have lunch with one or two of his friends, then come home. I should have known that teachers have a fondness for free slaves. I should have remembered that I had never known a teacher in my school years who cleaned their own blackboard duster, picked anything up off the floor and had used children to fetch and carry all manner of things.

We piled onto the bus in the school parking lot, where I discovered another phenomenon I had forgotten. Children on buses are loud enough to be heard in outer space.

At the reptile park, in the shade of the giant dinosaur, with the blinding sun peeling layers from my eyes, I waited to be told what to do, something I hadn't been very good at while a primary school student myself.

I was allocated ten eight-year-old boys by a vengeful teacher who immediately disappeared with several small girls who seemed to worship her and hang on her every word like tiny sycophants.

Ten. Ye gods, what would I do with ten of them? The boys were fidgeting and scuffing their feet like a herd of wildebeests anxious to cross a river. I wondered how many directions ten small boys could go off in. I could so easily lose control, so I decided the best thing to do was to keep moving and sound as though I knew exactly what I was doing and where I was going.

I followed the vengeful teacher and her queue of duckling-girls. That took care of the "where". Until my lot were sidetracked and the teacher disappeared around a corner with no thought of my peril. The rest of the day can best be described as damage control, where I lost the plot that I'd never had, cursed all teachers, and all eight-year-old boys.

I didn't know all eight of the boys, but I recognised one with growing horror. Robby Mansfield. The only child to have had so many meetings with the teachers and the principal that his imminent expulsion from the school had been discussed. He had started a fire in class, assaulted other boys and slapped a teacher. Apparently, his vocabulary was enhanced by profuse swearing.

Robby whooped with joy at the sight of so many dangerous creatures. He found a huge stick and poked it into every cage and enclosure. I yelled. Gerard stared at me. This was a sound he had never heard. He was stunned at first, then impressed. I wanted the ground to open up and swallow me. I was never going to survive this day. I would be held accountable for the actions of a miniature hoodlum.

Then I gave up, deciding that if approached, I would point at the vengeful teacher who had set me up with the little monster.

I snatched the stick from Robby and threw it over my shoulder. He found a bigger one, poked it down into a possum enclosure with a narrow opening. A cunning possum, seeing the possibility of freedom, lost no time in racing up the stick and off. The right thing to do would have been to notify the park rangers. I did no such thing. I had ten boys going in at least five directions.

I shuddered through the spider milking where the boys were on their best behaviour for the park attendant. I may have closed my eyes. A girl can only cope with so many flashback-nightmares.

I masterfully tried to shorten the circuit around the park by avoiding the loop that went by the snake pits. But the boys saw through my strategy, and led by the intrepid Robby, they leaned into the snake enclosure with the kind of glee I had only seen at birthday parties. I nearly passed out when Robby found yet another stick and proceeded to poke. I didn't look. I didn't see. I walked away. Off down the track, hoping to find an exit, the empty waiting bus, and my sanity. Robby caught up at the crocodile enclosure, where he abandoned his stick-poking to throw rocks while attempting to gain a better height by climbing the fence.

'Don't do th...' I began, then I remembered Natural Selection and walked away.

Back at the bus, the vengeful teacher looked as fresh as a daisy, and I looked anything but. I wondered what had happened to the possum and the snakes, and hoped the crocodile hadn't been so enraged that it decided to attack the staff.

Robby sat behind me on the bus.

I grabbed the little monster by the hand and dumped him on the vengeful teacher, telling her I had a headache that would split bricks, and if there were any reports from the park of escaping creatures, it had nothing to do with me.

A family remade

I met Adam, my second husband, at a party for church singles. A handsome man, softly spoken with a shy demeanour, he seemed to be everything my first husband had lacked. Adam fell in love quickly, then out of it again, often giving me an update of his devotion as a percentage. A pattern that continued.

A step-father

One day, not long before we were married, Adam took eleven-year-old Gerard to the local creek for a swim. They found a rope swing and proceeded to do what boys do. When they arrived home, Adam was covered in bruises and scratches from head to toe. Gerard, who was a master at saying nothing, said nothing, and said it very well.

Adam treated us to an extremely lengthy account of how it was the tree's fault, an epistle that Gerard and I found very amusing. For a long time after, we would indulge in lengthy discussions, accompanied by much hilarity and snorting, on how the tree had shifted. Various hurricane-inspired conspiracy theories were developed, much to Adam's disgust and disdain. He would respond, 'You people don't know what you are talking about.' We never did.

Adam had grown up with a violent, drunken father, and his endeavours to outrun this heritage softened my heart. However, others were less impressed.

My darling Uncle Gordon refused to come to our wedding because of Adam's inconsistency. When I told Gerard that I was marrying Adam, he threw his teddy bears on the floor. He had always been a serious child, and I thought it was a matter of time before he accepted Adam.

I later realised the profound implication of this action. It was as articulate as an eleven-year-old boy could be.

At the wedding, a girl I had babysat as a teenager sang, 'Sometimes when we touch the honesty's too much'.

A poignant foreshadowing…

My best friend was handed a microphone at the wedding reception and said, 'If Linda had listened to me, we couldn't be here.'

Adam thanked her for letting him off lightly.

Adam's piece de resistance, however, was when he blew up my laundry. This took place several months after we were married. Adam had a favourite shirt he wore when helping 'fix' his brother-in-law's car. I don't think the car ever went again.

The shirt had so much grease on it that it was hard to tell what its previous colour had been, but he was not impressed when he found it in the rubbish bin, relegated there by me. So after a little bit of preaching about my laundry skills and general lack of respect for a man's property, he proceeded to use kerosene to get the stains out. Kerosene, he proclaimed, had unrivalled effectiveness to remove grease.

He then found he couldn't get the kerosene out. By this time, a whole load of washing had also been contaminated by the kerosene. After a bit more lecturing, Adam moved on to remove the kerosene from the shirt by using petrol as a, God help me, 'solvent'. He carried the jerry can full of petrol into the laundry and rinsed the whole sink full of clothes with it before pouring copious amounts of sudsy water over them in an attempt to, yes, get the petrol out.

I walked into the room as he was putting the whole sorry mess into the washing machine. On this occasion, I took a leaf out of Gerard's book and said nothing. After all, I had heard enough lectures for one day, including one, ironically enough, that even centred on Adam's expertise and experience as a Volunteer Fire Fighter in Victoria.

The washing machine began to fill, and for once in my life, I decided that discretion was the better part of valour and walked out of the room.

The washing machine started. The electricity sparked. And the laundry went off like a bomb. A fireball followed me out. He was dead, I knew it. I did what all practical women do in such a crisis. I screamed. I was immobilised by fear. Not Adam, however. After what seemed like hours but was probably only a few seconds, he streaked out of the laundry, yelling instructions like a warlord. Still numb with shock, I didn't understand a word he was yelling. He ran outside. He ran inside. He ran outside again. He ran back into the laundry where there was a nice combination of fire, electricity and water. He grabbed the jerry can, by this time with flames coming out of the top, and ran outside again. Obviously not content with his earlier near brush with death, he was determined to put paid to his existence by carrying a potential bomb supplied by the huge, lethal, flaming jerry can.

Meanwhile, the fracas attracted the children, Gerard, and Adam's daughter.

Gerard frowned, went outside to the meter box and turned the electricity off, something his clever step-father hadn't thought to do. Gerard then went into the laundry, where the flames had died down and were confined to the laundry tub. He threw a blanket over the flames and wandered back out to the main event of chaos.

Fearing deep burns on Adam's legs, I ordered him into a cold bath and then asked the kids to go to the neighbours' to get ice or anything frozen to add to the bath. There sat Adam, naked from the waist down, in the bath with broccoli, peas and raspberries, still able to sound forth on how we were all useless, prone to panic and had no idea what to do in a crisis.

Adam's legs looked suspiciously red, so I phoned the ambulance. The ambulance arrived. The officer with a rounded girth and bunched muscles crossed his arms and surveyed a half-naked Adam in the frozen soup bath. The fire department and police weren't needed as Gerard had thrown a blanket over the fire.

'Well, sunshine, what have we here?' asked the ambulance officer, with a decided smirk wreathing his face.

Adam informed him that he was fine, "thank you very much, " and he could not comprehend what had possessed his overreacting wife to phone them.

'Stand up and show me sunshine.'

Sunshine stood up. He was not so fine without the ice water. His red, angry legs wobbled as the blow torch effect of the burns set in.

'I think we'd better take you to the doctor, sunshine.'

Sunshine went.

On the way out the door, I suggested that he might want to accept pain relief. Adam pompously informed me that he would need no such thing. He was not a drug addict like me who took pain relief for migraines or any old disc pain. I was told later that by the time Adam got to the surgery, he had howled like a baby and begged for pethidine. The ambulance officer wouldn't give it to him because of his pompous rant at me. The doctor had pity on him and gave it to him.

He was admitted to the local private hospital for observation and treatment of his burns and stayed for over a week. After daily dressings and assessment, when the blisters subsided, it was determined that his burns were 'second degree' and not full thickness. He had narcotic injections several times, and no one called *him* a drug addict. He took the opportunity in his new calm horizontal state to read a heavy tome by Paul Tournier, the French psychiatrist and theologian and claimed to benefit greatly from his enforced stay with the faint suggestion that it had 'elevated his thinking'.

I liked him very much in his new mellow state. Initially, I didn't want to worry him by discussing all the cleaning up and expenses, but his newfound peace and euphoria soon began to annoy me, so I told him about *all* of the work and expenses we were facing. 'It's only money,' he said, floatingly from his lofty vantage point. This waffle from the same man who once lectured me for more than an hour on the economic advantages and costs of purchasing the 500g Weet-Bix packet, which was the only size he would endorse.

The insurance company paid immediately without a qualm. Apparently, Adam wasn't the only moron to accomplish this feat. Years later, the same insurance company refused to pay for a bathroom destroyed by water damage from leaking pipes inside the wall cavity, which was a building fault. They were prepared to fund an act of idiocy, but not a plumbing mistake that wasn't our fault.

A Barrel Chest

Gerard had "round shoulders" and was very self-conscious about it. One doctor suggested I bandage a ruler across his back to encourage better posture. I didn't.

A physiotherapist suggested some exercises to correct it. Others thought he spent too much time reading and using the computer.

I didn't realise the depth of Gerard's discomfort until much later, but I could see his spirits sink a little lower each time someone commented on his round shoulders. He found it hard to express his feelings and often resisted my attempts to get him to open up.

When we relocated to Coffs Harbour, the curvature seemed to be getting worse, so I took him to a new doctor, a straightforward and immensely qualified man, who had seen a lot of life. He knew instinctively how to approach a sensitive teenage boy.

'Is there anyone with a barrel chest in the family?' he asked.

'*Oh yes!*' was Gerard's excited reply. My uncle, his beloved great-uncle Gordon, had a *huge* chest.

The doctor delivered the good news. Gerard was developing a barrel chest, a large chest structure of the type last seen on Mike Tyson.

A flush of awe passed over Gerard's face when he thought of the big man who had been a medic in the 4th Field Ambulance during

WWII, one who had marched the Kokoda trail and taught him how to mow lawns and care for machinery.

On the way home in the car, Gerard spoke of his fears and his relief in an excited, machine-gun fashion. These words showed the depth of his anguish. He had renewed optimism. His life looked instantly brighter. He had hoped that his problem could be fixed, but had learned he didn't need fixing at all.

Sure enough, he developed the biggest chest we had seen in a long time. Plus the strength of ten strong men to go with it. A lung capacity that impressed his dive instructor. He could finally shed the hated taunts of his classmates, crop his curls deathly short and scare the pants off anyone he wanted to just by looking like a surly bouncer. And they never knew he was as gentle as his bear of an uncle had been.

"That kid is lazy!"

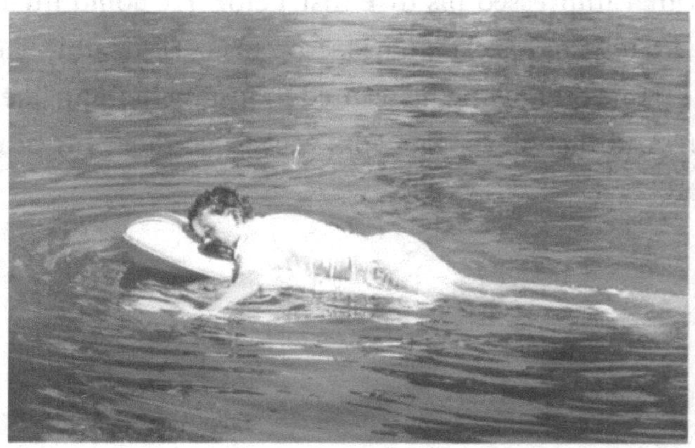

After the wedding, it wasn't long before it became apparent that Adam did not hold any affection for his new stepson. Adam perceived Gerard's silence as insolence and was irked at Gerard's ability to do well at school without even glancing at homework.

Gerard's effortless prowess with computers and technology further fuelled Adam's ire.

However, it was Gerard's place in my affection that bruised Adam's frail ego the most. Gerard was openly affectionate, something missing from Adam's DNA.

Only three months into the marriage, a group of us went to play tennis at the local school courts. Gerard owned a tennis racquet and so did I, although I had no intention of joining the fray with Adam and his competitive relatives.

Gerard and one of the relatives' sons found a court and started to have fun with our racquets.

A kerfuffle arose in the adults' court. I was knitting, or some other inane activity, to allay the boredom of watching persons of intense focus hit a ball back and forth while arguing every toss. The noise level rose, and then it was on.

Adam lost his temper and started yelling.

It took me a while to work out what had caused his anger and just which person or inanimate object had raised his ire. Apparently, the adults were one racquet short.

Adam demanded that the two teen boys give up a racquet to the adults because "adults came first".

'No,' I said. 'That's rubbish. They're my racquets. I brought them, provided them. With foresight, I might add. If the "adults" failed to bring enough racquets to play with, then that's their fault.'

Adam stormed off.

In the car.

Down the road.

Thankfully, the tennis courts were on the street where we lived in my house, so the journey for Gerard and me, and Adam's daughter was mercifully short.

When we arrived back at the house, Adam was packing. He had borrowed his mother's trailer and was filling it with fervour. Suitcases came out of the house with lids half-closed.

Adam yelled at his daughter to pack her things. She didn't know where to put her cases because Adam was loading two baby goats into the trailer, kids that he had acquired days earlier and had been given the names of Abraham and Joseph.

'Be a lot quieter without those two bloody animals,' said Gerard.

Adam's destination was his mother's house on the other side of town. She phoned me and said, 'Don't worry, love. He'll be back.'

'What if I don't want him back?' I said, thinking that she might be okay with pendulum husbands, but I was not.

'Oh dear, love.'

Sadly, he did come back, of course. However, there was one bright spot on the horizon. Adam left Abraham and Joseph with his mother's ewe, unimaginatively named "Lamb Lamb".

One day, out with Adam, the car broke down. We were walking to get help, always a doubtful enterprise with Adam.

As a teenager, Gerard was starving. I spied a Pizza Hut and my stomach growled in sympathy. I can't remember why, but none of us was wearing shoes. Adam was horrified at the thought of going inside. Gerard said nothing. He knew I would go inside in the face of any opposition, even if it was just for him.

'I'm not going *in that place* to make a complete fool of myself!' Adam said.

'Suit yourself.' I headed toward the entry.

'What? ... You're not serious... you can't...'

I turned to Adam. 'If you walk like you are wearing shoes, no one will look at your feet. It's the Pizza Hut, not the Ritz. And quite honestly, people are NOT that interested in what other people do unless it gets in the way of what they want.'

Gerard and I went into the restaurant. We were getting stuck into pizza when Adam sheepishly wandered in, high-stepping like a Greek soldier, his lack of shoes obvious to all.

We spent one holiday in Manila. Not the Asian destination that springs to mind, but a town not far from Tamworth. Adam was a fitness devotee, the likes of whom had never been seen in **my** family.

He set about swimming back and forth across the river with great enthusiasm.

Gerard, on the other hand, carried his inflatable bed up to the bridge, where he placed it in the river and let the water carry him back to where he started.

This activity incensed Adam. 'That kid is bone lazy,' he said, not seeming to notice that Gerard jogged up to the bridge every time.

Sport

Gerard never really embraced the concept or action of Sport. I couldn't blame him. I was not a good example. After primary school, where I enjoyed Rounders and cricket with the boys, I had seriously gone off the whole thing. Mainly because I was rubbish at it.

In high school, our whole Year 12 class enjoyed playing hockey with our Maths/Science teacher, whose antics entertained us immensely. It didn't matter that I was still rubbish.

Gerard, on the other hand, was good. Really good. Surprising, as he never engaged in sport of any kind. He had swimming lessons, and he rode a bike everywhere. That must have counted for something.

At one primary swimming carnival, Gerard actually competed in one race; at least he started. He had been seriously bribed by Nannie. However, on the day Gerard was swimming, Nannie ran along the edge of the pool, in front of the whole school and assembled parents, yelling, 'Come on, Gerard, Go, Gerard.'

Gerard went. He came straight out of the pool and walked home.

Gerard's attitude was more than a disappointment to his sport-mad step-father, Adam, who threw himself into any sporting activity until he needed his Ventolin inhaler.

As headmaster of a one-teacher school in Coffs Harbour, Adam was involved in goading all the students into competing at the Combined Schools Sports Carnival. Five small schools had combined for the event.

Adam couldn't cope with Gerard refusing to participate. He asked, then went straight to threats, pouting, lectures on his reputation and finally begged Gerard to compete in at least one event.

Gerard, who hardly ever gave in to pressure of any kind, reluctantly agreed, 'Alright, ONE.'

The 100-metre sprint was agreed upon. Adam would save face by having his step-son participate. How would it look if he couldn't manage his own family?

Gerard lined up with the other twelve-year-olds, in his daggy sneakers, looking mutinous and pissed off.

The other kids leaned forward. One of them was a track and field star who hoped for State glory.

Gerard hoped to shrink into the crowd and for the day to be over.

The starter's gun went off.

Gerard loped. He didn't appear to be putting in the effort required for any kind of success.

Gerard flew across the grass and came first.

The crowd cheered. Gerard cringed and walked over to me.

Adam was astonished. I was astonished. The whole crowd roared. Where had this protégé come from? This star?

Adam was thrilled, believing that this stunning success would please Gerard so much that he would now want to enter every event.

Gerard did not want to enter any other event and regretted

agreeing to this event.

When the ribbon ceremony occurred at the end of the race, Gerard refused to go and collect his first prize ribbon, so his red-faced step-father had to go up and get it.

Gerard shoved it in a pocket.

Adam pleaded for Gerard to go in the relay race. Success was now assured with a kid like this. Adam hissed and threatened, to no avail.

No, Gerard did not want to compete in the relay race.

Gerard wanted everyone to stop looking at him, talking about him and pressuring him. He hadn't meant to win the race.

I must admit that I was disappointed. I felt that sport was more socially important for boys and didn't want Gerard to face the teasing of his peers. But Gerard didn't care one jot if his peers teased him.

Later, when Gerard was in Year 10, I renewed my hope that he would get involved in one sport or another. After all, it was necessary for the School Certificate.

Gerard promised me that he would sign up for a sport. When he came home that afternoon, I asked him if he had signed on.

'Yes, mother.'

'What did you sign up for?'

'Board games.'

Pedant

Some people only see one point of view, so they come across as thinking themselves superior to the rest of us. This makes them sound pedantic, probably because they are pedantic. They make good headmasters. I know this because I married one. A pedant and a headmaster.

Adam was never wrong. Lesser mortals were referred to as 'you people'. 'You people' didn't know what they were talking about. 'You people' couldn't see something right in front of their eyes. I can remember listening in awe to his many finely delivered lectures. With his towering height and his sportsman's physique, he was impressive, before he spoke, that is. He had such an air of confident authority and such a booming voice that many people would have believed him if he said he, and not Moses, had led the children of Israel across the Red Sea. I tried not to question or argue with him in public. I didn't try hard enough.

Once, Adam had a three-day argument with Gerard about Nebuchadnezzar, the Persian King in the Old Testament who lived like an animal and survived for nine years by eating grass. Gerard suggested that it was not possible for a human being to do this and that the lesson the Bible was trying to teach had nothing to do with the ingestion of plant cellulose, but something else altogether.

Gerard's opinion was not welcome, and Adam proceeded to tell him at great length how wrong he was. As usual, this involved long and pedantic searches through the encyclopedia and any other resource that either of them saw fit to come up with.

Gerard was highly amused and entertained with this diversion from all the other boredoms of life and entered into it with zeal. Adam was not amused *or* entertained and entered into it with altogether different zeal.

Adam ended with his favourite statement, 'I know I'm right', and Gerard fell back on his usual ploy and said nothing, that is, until he remarked much later, 'he's an idiot'. The idiot could thereafter be goaded on this subject at the drop of a hat.

Whenever we travelled, if Adam needed to stop at the service station to use the bathroom, he insisted that *everyone* go. He would wake everyone up and demand that we all get out and go to the toilet. This did not go down well with the teenagers in the car. Or with me.

I would either salute him, dance on the spot, or call him Daddy. This did not go down well with Adam, but it brought a wide smile to Gerard, who enjoyed any sign of a light moment amid Adam's tyranny.

After we were married, Adam was in the kitchen conducting whispered crisis talks with his daughter while staring into the open fridge. Deliberations continued, and even though I knew the only result would be condemnation, I stepped into the fray and enquired politely as to the cause of the whispered conference.

Ever one to jump to the worst-case scenario, I assumed that a two-foot rat had crawled into the fridge and died.

It appeared, however, that the margarine wasn't flat. It had seen better days, and whoever had used it last had gouged and dug rather than horizontally scraped.

This was a whole new world of life requirements for me. I tried to understand; after all, love me, love my obsession. I was given a pompous lecture on the necessity of flat margarine and the techniques for maintaining it, with Adam's daughter nodding calm agreement.

I kept a straight face, for a day at least, and then a wicked demon on my shoulder whispered in my ear.

A day later, I collapsed in the kitchen, hyperventilating.

They all came running. The all-wise, all-knowing headmaster, the disapproving daughter, and Gerard, my smirking son, sensing some free entertainment. At least the boy knew me.

When Adam and his daughter saw me lying, having paroxysms on the floor, gasping and panting, they politely asked if I needed an ambulance.

I panted, 'I can't cope.'

'What? Why?'

'The margarine is still not flat!'

Gerard grinned and said, 'Good one, Mum', but Adam and his daughter walked off in stony silence.

A second brother

Adam knew I wanted another child when he met me. I finally fell pregnant two years after the marriage.

Bronson was born, not wide-eyed with knowing concern like Gerard. This babe was all bunched up and squinting, yowling and yawning. His mouth always seeking. His head turned to find me. Curving his body into mine, murmuring soft kitten noises.

When Bronson was only a few hours old, he grasped his big brother's finger and didn't let go.

Gerard was fourteen. He leant his rangy body over the clear Perspex crib. The blistering sun bathed them in a golden summer glow, framed through a square window overlooking gum trees. I watched them reverently whispering, 'my two sons, my two sons' knowing I would remember that day, that moment, forever.

Gerard stood stock-still in wonder, holding the hand of the newest human being he had ever seen with a commitment that said "I am here for you". Gerard had worried about me, having heard stories of my medical dramas with his first brother. On this day of his second brother's birth he forgave me for risking my life for this child, this brother.

A voice said the baby has some uncle's chin.

Gerard was astonished and muttered—'Frigging baby doesn't have a chin!'

Because Adam's work responsibilities didn't allow for any time off, he stated that he would not be taking any paternity leave. I hadn't really expected him to. I was surprised he had even heard of it but one of the guys from church had asked him about it. This made Adam feel that I might need some assistance after giving birth by caesarean. He came home from church and said, 'Gerard can stay home and look after you and the baby. It's not as if he learns anything at school anyway.'

Gerard and I exchanged surprised looks. I feigned opposition to the idea and then gracefully accepted Adam's superior knowledge.

Gerard stepped up as if he had been doing precisely this all his life, and with calm, patient grace. He rinsed dirty nappies on the back lawn with the hose, then washed them in the machine before putting them in the drier. He folded them carefully. He changed Bronson's nappies, cooing at his tiny brother. He made me toast and Vegemite, and cups of tea. He didn't need to do any of it because I had coped alone when he was a newborn. I grew tired of Adam's mandate to use cloth nappies and bought disposables. That ended the backyard shenanigans.

Gerard seemed to know instinctively how to treat his brother. He would place Bronson on his chest and lie in front of the television where Bronson slept soundly, never reacting to the noise of the cartoons or whatever else Gerard was watching. This infuriated Adam so Gerard omitted these activities when Adam was home.

No one else could settle Bronson who jerked awake whenever he was put down to sleep, in the cot, in the bassinet, or in the pram, unless he had the comfort of a body.

As Bronson grew older, he crawled around in Gerard's room, throwing things on the floor, something that amused Gerard. His brother was welcome anywhere.

Gerard writes about Bronson

Infants have the most intoxicating ability to both amaze and be amazed simultaneously. Things you can watch a child do for hours would bore you to tears coming from an adult. Imagine a co-worker telling you a story during a lunch break about a fascinating insect he saw on the weekend.

They proceed in great detail and eloquence describing every sensation and emotion they felt when this tiny red creature with black spots crawled over their finger in the park. They relate to you the sorrow they felt when it flew away and the frustration of not being able to find it again. But it was ok because the journey to find that small insect led them to what has to be the most fantastic piece of wood in the whole world, it was shaped like…

And it's about here in the story where my response would be 'So you found a lady bug and stick right?' It's just not that interesting, but having said that, when I was about sixteen I watched my two year old brother play with bits of nature in a park for a good three hours one day. His reaction to the world and his own little first time experience was captivating.

Another time it was a ping pong ball. Picture a warm Sunday afternoon when you really can't think of a single reason to stop lying on the floor. Bronson was about 14 months old and sitting in his bouncinette. I found a ping pong ball and on a whim put it in my mouth and blew it upwards. As it flew up into the air it made a loud 'pop' noise.

If I had been alone in the room this might have kept me away from the television for no more than a few pops, however Bronson found it insanely funny, I don't mean I just got a chuckle from him—he laughed as hard as a baby can without needing to be changed afterwards.

And it was one of those laughs young kids get when they haven't really decided how they are going to laugh later in life and are still making up their minds on how it should be done. His enthusiasm and his reaction to what he found to be just the funniest thing ever just poured out of him.

I didn't find his reaction funny, his laugh wasn't particularly infectious. But it did make me happy, tears in the eyes happy. Having both just had such fun with such a simple thing I did it again, and again and again. It never got old for him, and his joy never got old for me. I'm not sure how long I 'popped' that ball but I had sore lips and I'm sure his stomach muscles got a workout too. The rest of the people in the house got tired of it long before we did.

I guess I just wanted to connect with that tiny person, our experiences at that point were too different for there to be any real common ground or more accurately shared communication, so when I did find something we had in common or even just got a familiar reaction to something I did I loved it. Here was a small person who couldn't understand a word I said, couldn't speak English, had no manners, was a total mooch and when presented with my hand only really wanted to suck on the end of my finger.

And yet he was still the coolest little person I'd met.

A step-father: Opus of Rage

I

Adam waits in tense silence, hearing the stumbling footfall on the doorstep, then muffled cursing as a key jars in the lock. His father is home.

Adam is fourteen years old, his lanky body taut as he slides from his bed to stand at the bedroom door, his head bent, leaning into the darkness. He stretches muscles that are tight from helping his mother with her evening cleaning job. It keeps food on the table.

The sound of grinding gears woke him minutes earlier. He is a light sleeper, a restless one, with the honed instincts of a soldier. Attune to the night, he listens. He fights an electric prickle of anxiety, waiting for the signs that are precursors to violence.

Violence threads through his days, even while his athletic body finds release in sport, basketball, soccer, and cross-country. Violence taints his nights, even the quiet ones—those somnolent stretches of peace. Because there is always a shadow. A shadow that thunders, retreats and returns.

Adam winces at the sound of clattering in the kitchen. He moans, tonight will not be one of those nights his father passes out on the couch. *Stay in your room, Mum*—his silent prayer. He does not understand why she pleads, placates, or sometimes fights back.

There is no way to comprehend why the walls of this house shape the construct of the most dangerous place he has ever known.

The police come often. His father hurls abuse at them with democratic ease.

A scraping, shuffling noise tells him one of the younger ones has been woken and is going to the toilet. His hands clench. He hears his mother's soft voice to the child, and prays his father won't hear. In vain.

It begins—the dense drama that is family life.

'Why can't you make those children obey you?'—the opening prelude to the opus of rage.

Adam steps into the hallway. Menace radiates from the man in front of him; he is both stranger and father. Fast, angry and drunk, his father strikes. The younger children are all awake now, screaming, whimpering, clawing at their mother's nightie.

Adam towers over his stocky father. Once his mere presence was enough to stop the onslaught, but not anymore. Once he merely protected the others, now he is aggressor.

'You're as bad as me,' his father roars.

In the morning, they will work side by side, hammering, planning, building. Each in their own silence.

Adam will respect and honour his father. In the morning. But tonight he is measuring blow for blow.

Adam vows, I will never be like you.

II

Adam paces the upstairs kitchen. He's stressed. It's been a tough week. No one seems to understand the pressure of trying to teach dozens of kids, no one in this house anyway. Not the people under his own roof. Not the woman he married after his divorce, the one who soothes and coddles her own son, as well as the baby she has borne to him. The son he dreamed of, a son to carry his name.

His wife is breastfeeding the baby now, cooing and caressing the infant's downy head. He doesn't know why but this affection grates. 'I wish you wouldn't demand feed,' he says, his voice rising. 'I don't agree with it. *On demand*, who does that? Don't you see? Kids who are demand fed are spoiled.'

Adam fumes. He should be the head of the house. And as for that boy, *her* fourteen-year-old son, the kid shows *no* respect. To anyone. The boy's surly silences infuriate, prickle and crawl under his skin, eating at him, taunting him. He would rather open rebellion, heated exchanges than this, this voiceless insolence. This arrogant obedience. He approaches her, his anger fermenting. 'I sent that kid down to tidy the garage. What's taking him so long?'

'Maybe he doesn't know where to put your tools, your things,' she says. 'It's chaos down there.'

Adam stabs at her with a finger. 'I'm too busy to run a house as well as a school.' His voice is gritty, resentful. He stands at the top of the stairs and calls the boy. 'Makes my blood boil,' he mutters, clenching his teeth. He is greeted with silence, then a shuffling sound, feet scraping. The sounds of reluctance. The stairwell amplifies the sound. He waits. His blood is heating. She's oblivious, sitting in the lounge that backs onto the stair railing. Still petting the baby. She'll ruin the kids, both of them. Turn them into sappy, spoiled brats.

He watches as the boy begins his slow ascent. He launches into a blistering tirade. The boy says nothing, not even when he is standing on the step below him.

Adam lands a full-body blow that spills the boy down the stairs. He follows, roaring and punching. Then kicking as the boy lies still. He rains blows, vision blurred, control gone. 'Why don't you fight like a man?' he rages. The boy whispers, *I will never be like you.*

Adam hears his wife scream, an endless piercing that fractures the air. He runs back up the stairs to her. 'I only stopped hitting *that boy* because I heard you scream and thought you'd dropped MY son!' She freezes. He rants. He speaks of righteous indignation, of respect, of obedience. Then he leaves, taking the phone and the car.

Placing the baby down with care, she runs down the stairs, heart pounding, calling her son's name. Unaware that she had screamed, she wonders if her son is alive. She finds him, pale, cold and bleeding. Bruised and crouching. She weeps. She weeps for wounds she can never heal, for a heart that cannot be unbroken. For a son who will wear the scars of battle. From a man she brought into his life. She weeps for a son who will cross the bridge to manhood with a tainted, seared psyche. She attends to him. She finds a public phone. They don't take teenage boys at the refuge. It's a new town, and she knows no one. Isolation and fear claw at her stomach. She moves in a fog.

When Adam returns, he is still fermenting. He strides through the house with primal rage. He is livid. They have no idea how far they've pushed him, what they have made him become. He demands respect. She pleads softly to take the boys and stay with her mother, 'just for a few days, to let everyone heal, get past things.' He spins to face her. 'Walk out that door, and I'll take my son, and you'll never see him again.' The air is taut with menace. He turns to glare at the boy who is standing in the corner, then slides his eyes to her. 'You won't find me, but I'll find you. Then no one else will find you.'

Gerard retreats. It's a habit he will take into manhood.

Gerard vows. I will never be like you.

Escape to Nan

I was shocked and distressed by Adam's treatment of Gerard. Adam's rage continued. I stood between him and Gerard, constantly vigilant. I kept Bronson close, his bassinette by the bed at night, in my arms during the day. I desperately wanted to leave, but I was paralysed by Adam's threats to take Bronson away, where I would never see him again if I left. Every day, Adam unplugged the phone and took it with him. He kept an eye on the car keys, making sure I couldn't have them. There were no mobile phones in 1993.

We had just moved to Toowoomba. I knew no one. It had been only a couple of months since Bronson's birth and my C-section. I had no money. I walked to a pay phone up the road and phoned a women's shelter, but was told that I couldn't bring a 14-year-old boy there.

I had no hope that the police would intervene and help. In retrospect, I should have phoned them, but I was afraid of the repercussions if I was forced to return to the house with the boys. Where would they put me? Where could I go? Could I report something when Gerard refused?

I asked Adam if I could visit my mother – 'just to let us all get over this', but Adam repeated his threats. He phoned his mother, who told him, 'Don't let her go, she'll never come back.'

My mother was travelling in New Zealand. I couldn't have gone to her.

I told Adam that I was taking Gerard out of school for a fortnight and organising a counsellor. I was adamant that this was necessary. School wouldn't accept an absence without medical verification. Adam reluctantly agreed.

I sat with Gerard. 'If he is close to God, I never want to be,' he said. 'I don't know if I can ever forgive him.'

'I don't either,' I said.

When we attended church for the first time since moving to Toowoomba, I was thrilled to find a friend from my school days. She observed Adam and said to me, 'After that pointing finger comes the fist.'

I was amazed that she had assessed Adam so quickly. She introduced me to a woman who worked in the hospital with domestic violence victims, and she recommended a psychologist, a big bloke who had been in the Australian Navy. A real man.

The first counsellor, an older woman, hadn't connected with Gerard at all. He felt defeated.

I told Gerard about the new guy. He shrugged. 'I won't go,' he said.

'I can't keep you out of school if you don't have a medical certificate.'

'Okay.'

Gerard went. I later learned that he didn't speak during the first session. The psychologist knew exactly how to handle this, and this new situation was a perfect fit.

Gerard told me that he wanted to leave and live with his grandmother. I couldn't fight that. He deserved peace. He didn't choose this marriage, this abuse and chaos.

I watched Gerard leave, with his hat pulled down over his eyes, sitting in the bus, head down. I watched the bus until it was out of sight, then went back to the house and cried all day.

I missed him profoundly and looked forward to our phone calls. I cried in the garage, hoping Adam wouldn't hear me.

On arriving at his grandmother's, Gerard wasted no time getting into trouble, which was painfully predictable.

He talked Nannie into getting him a motorbike. I was appalled. He was fifteen. Mum lied and said it was 'all in bits – it'll take him forever to put it together'. However, Gerard was out and about in no time. The bike had not been in "bits" at all.

Gerard found that the friends he had before were happy to accept him back into their fold.

Gerard set about frustrating his teachers with a lack of interest and cooperation. Nana, who knew the Principal well, went back and forth to the school and phoned me to 'make the kid do what I tell him.'

Almost a year passed with Gerard doing as he pleased and Nannie wondering what to do. Gerard was happy. Happy to stay home on the computer. Happy to ride the motorbike. Happy to wander to school to see his mates almost every school day. Happy to visit them for computer nights. Happy and generally unconcerned about his grandmother's worries, unconcerned about his stupid mother's decision to stay with the idiot whom he had renamed "Dickhead.' Adam had gone from Dad to Dickhead.

A couple of Gerard's friends were honing their shoplifting skills.

Gerard, being a bit of a "know-it-all", was keen to show them that he could shoplift and be superior about it. He was. Gerard had always walked slowly, with purpose. He was incredibly aware of his surroundings, yet he looked as if he were just dreaming through life. Very soon, he outperformed the other boys, until…

A security guard met them in a shopping centre car park. When he accused one of the boys, two of the boys presented what they had taken. Gerard didn't, until he had to.

'How are you blokes getting home?' asked the security officer.

'Bus,' said Gerard.

'Car,' said one of the others. The security guard searched the car and found more. Quite a bit more.

They were duly arrested, and Nannie, beside herself with worry, phoned me and gave me their court date.

Adam, Bronson and I came down to attend the court. On the way in the car, I said to Gerard, 'Is this a career choice, or a phase?'

'Don't be silly, Mum,' he said. 'I'm a minor. I'm not taking this on when I'm an adult.'

'Good to know, Gerard.'

'I'm really good at it though,' he said with a wicked grin.

Gerard was wearing a T-shirt that had seen some wear.

Mum saw me giving the T-shirt a disapproving look. 'I couldn't get him to wear anything else.'

'Don't worry, Mum. It's not your responsibility.' How could I accuse her?

Mum held a folder. I asked for it.

There was a long list of charges. I was shocked.

'You said there was only one charge, Mum! There are thirteen.'

'I didn't look at it.'

'Thank goodness I organised a solicitor,' I said.

At the court, I realised that Gerard was the only one with a solicitor. One of the boys was facing other charges for another court appearance and his mother sat outside the court tatting, a complex craft that boggled my mind.

Gerard walked nonchalantly into the court with his hands in his pockets. The judge said, 'Take your hands out of your pockets, young man. You're in enough trouble. You will respect my court.'

My heart sank. Would I be visiting him in jail with a number on his chest?

Mum had been repeating to me that she couldn't take any more. I told her that she must tell Gerard, otherwise he would blame me, and I had centuries of blame and shame to live down already.

She muttered this news to Gerard outside the court with damp eyes and I hugged her. Gerard shrugged. It had been too good to last.

When he arrived back, Adam ranted, 'You will follow my rules as long as you are in this house.'

'It's Mum's house,' Gerard said calmly. I had paid for the house with a workers' compensation settlement.

Adam said nothing.

There had been a shift.

Game over

Awakened in the middle of the night, I squinted at the bedside clock. 2 am. Adam was yelling and punching the bed.

'I never wanted this house. I don't know why I let you choose it. You're happy. You with your renovating and planning, playing with that baby. But I'm not happy. I never wanted to live here.'

It was monumental nonsense. I had had my heart set on a modern house in town, walking distance to shops and close to Gerard's high school.

Adam had a form of relentless "persuasion" that involved resentment over what life had denied him and should now deliver. He had always wanted "a bit of land", although there was no evidence for efficient use of land in his recent or past history. He continued to take me to look over the property, chatting affably with the rotund real estate agent who declared that he had a personal interest in the property himself because it was "that good".

It was an isolated property in Drayton. No neighbours. Rough surfaces. Warped walls. 12 kilometres from Gerard's school.

Adam needed peace, a place where parents couldn't just drop in, although this had never happened. Adam wanted, Adam, Adam needed … I cringe as I write this. It's textbook coercive control.

I had grown to love the house. I had taken over organising the necessary renovations when Adam angrily gave up on the responsibility. I felt that I had been embraced by that house. The longer I lived there, the more I loved the house and the lifestyle it offered. I mistakenly thought Adam felt that way too. I was devastated to find that purchasing the rural dream did not make him happy. The anxieties and problems that had haunted our marriage returned to overthrow us. His anger was never far from the surface, sometimes distilled and often raging, but always wraithlike between us.

On a bright summer day, we returned to the house after shopping. Eighteen-month-old Bronson had done something to annoy his short-tempered father, so Adam decided to punish the toddler by 'leaving him in the car until the kid comes to his senses.'

I kept watch near the back door. Bronson was quiet. No crying or howling in protest, as expected by Adam. No evidence of understanding the consequences. Not a peep.

When Adam went back out to assess the toddler's penitence, he was disgusted to find that Bronson had eaten all his Butter Menthol soothers.

Adam was incensed. He dragged Bronson from the car by an arm, found a strip of ridged plastic and began to hit Bronson's bare legs. Bronson screamed. By the time I could intervene, Adam had Bronson in a cold bath, threatening to 'give him something to cry about.'

I confronted Adam.

'Get out, Linda. I'll deal with this.'

'I'm not moving an inch. Do you feel like a big man now? How does it feel to see fear in your son's eyes? What kind of man belts a toddler?'

Adam remonstrated, accusing me of soft love.

I said the one phrase I knew would hit home. 'Alright, Joe.'

Adam froze in shock. I had called him by his father's name.

He stood, shook water off his hands and stormed out of the bathroom.

Bronson had bruises on his legs. I didn't cover them when we visited friends. They knew instinctively what had happened.

Adam changed moods like the weather. One day, he started a rant about his claim to a generous nature. I was suffering from a case of the flu, with Gerard helping me.

Adam said, 'If I don't help you out, it's because you don't ask me. You can't blame me for that. That's on you. I can't fix what I don't know.'

I sighed, hoping for belated assistance of some kind. 'It would be lovely if you took Bronson for a while,' I said.

Adam fussed about, then put Bronson in the car before I could protest. I had only wanted him to take Bronson in the stroller for a long walk, but I heard the car roar off. Adam was angry. Fear grabbed me. It was 9 am. I hoped Adam would return soon, but as the day went on, I became more worried.

I paced. I couldn't rest. Gerard comforted me.

At 4 pm, I phoned the police. They said there was nothing they could do unless someone had come to harm.

I was distraught. I phoned the friends who had seen the bruises. They gave me the contact details for a solicitor. I phoned him.

Adam finally returned. He refused to hand Bronson over to me, even though Bronson was fractious and reaching for me. Adam headed for the bed with Bronson, saying they both needed sleep.

I knew Bronson wouldn't settle. I also knew that Adam would soon run out of patience. I gathered Bronson's nappy bag and a few things into the kitchen and said to Gerard, 'When you see me heading for the door, walk out before me.'

Gerard nodded, ever watchful.

Bronson called for me. He wriggled and resisted his father's hold.

'Go on then, go to your mother.' Adam released Bronson and turned over to sleep.

Quickly and quietly, we left. I had somewhere to go. Friends to protect me, merely by their presence. Somewhere to be safe. Where there was a phone. I had a solicitor. I had saved a little money from dressmaking and hidden it from Adam.

That evening, Adam phoned and asked when I was coming home.

'I'm not,' I said, 'ever. I am done. This is over.'

Adam walked to the friends' home and blustered. He grabbed Bronson. Gerard walked over to him and stood, blocking his exit. Everything had changed. There was a real man in the house.

At the court, when interviewed, I told a policeman that Adam had threatened to kill me. 'They all say that,' said the officer.

It wasn't safe to move back into the house, so I rented a flat. Other friends from church helped shift the furniture we needed.

One of the men, who was often at our house and played tennis with Adam, commandeered a Ute and filled the tray with furniture. He packed the huge, heavy dining table that Adam had made. It was in two separate pieces. Stem and tabletop. Adam bragged to anyone who would listen that he made that table.

When the guys arrived at the flat, one said, 'I have bad news. The tabletop fell out of the Ute while we were driving here, and the last we saw of it, it was wobbling down the main street, weaving through the traffic before crashing into a ditch. It's wrecked. Looks like a shark attacked it. We didn't want to go back for it. Sorry.'

I laughed. Gerard came. He laughed. I told the story of the table's preciousness. We all laughed.

A week after we moved into the flat, Adam phoned, furious. He said he had a jerry can of petrol and was coming around to blow himself up.

I ran around the house, frantic to leave for somewhere safe.

'What's wrong, Mum?' Gerard asked.

I told him. He ran to the kitchen.

'What are you doing, Gerard?'

'Looking for the matches. The idiot will forget to bring them.'

Manhood

Employment

Gerard had so many job changes that it seemed as if he couldn't persevere with anything. At seventeen, he started the theoretical portion of an electrical apprenticeship. This involved a 45-minute car journey to a Newcastle suburb that didn't have public transport. I drove him there and picked him up after work.

With electrical theory under his belt, Gerard applied for an apprenticeship at the same place his grandfather and uncle had worked. He had also completed high school work experience there. One day, he came across his grandfather's signature on the machinery in the factory where his grandfather had worked for thirty-six years. At his new job, Gerard was supervised by two supervisors during his work experience. He got on well with one of the men, who shared his temperament and focus and treated him as an equal. They both worked at a deliberate pace and complied with the rules.

However, Gerard didn't take the other supervisor's word on safety and checked everything himself, as he had been taught at TAFE. One day, the supervisor insisted that Gerard accept his word that the electricity had been turned off, but Gerard proved it was still live. This infuriated the supervisor, who accused Gerard of being a know-all.

Consequently, Gerard's application to that workplace was rejected. However, he still hoped to secure an electrical apprenticeship there and worked night shifts on the food production maintenance crew. The boss in this job made inappropriate remarks about me. Gerard gave him a brutal set-down, and so ended his job prospects at that workplace.

After that, Gerard was given the job of storeman. This was a perfect fit for an autistic person. The factory had experienced a serious problem with tools going missing, so a system requiring all tools to be signed out before use was implemented. This suited Gerard perfectly as he wouldn't allow anyone to circumvent the rules, even if they were high up in the company.

After Gerard came back to live with me, we talked about this job and how well it suited him. If only he had known about his autism then, it could have saved much angst later.

However, at the time, Gerard felt he should be more ambitious and achieve more, given his intellect and potential, so he applied for a job at a computer shop. It started well but soon became a disaster. Gerard lacked the charisma for retail and often told customers where they could get better quality or a better price. Nor did he dress with polish or have the kind of swagger deemed necessary for sales.

After trying various courses and jobs, Gerard drove trucks. He loved it. I didn't get it until we were moving house and Gerard drove the huge removal truck we hired. As I sat with him in the truck cab and saw him handle it so well, I understood his self-esteem and pride in his truck-driving job. He had no one to answer to, no one to tell him how to dress, how to behave, or what to say. He chatted happily to me as he drove.

While high-functioning autistic adults often have impressive skills, this does not necessarily increase an autistic person's chances of relating well in a job situation, as I have illustrated above. On the other hand, we find that many productive autistic people manage very well as sole business owners or in a small corner of a workplace with sympathetic autonomy.

For autistic adults, distress may be hard to perceive because they may be forthright and abrasive about what they see as injustices or changes to routine or expectations. They are often seen as outsiders who refuse or resist fitting in, in an age when teamwork is a byword for success. This affects their work and promotion prospects, even though they may have a significant contribution to offer. Rather than draw attention to their discomfort, they may prefer to leave jobs or situations where the level of adaptation required exceeds what they can handle. This is particularly true when they are confronted with multiple supervisors with different sets of regulations or levels of adherence to policy.

Additionally, frequent job changes compound feelings of failure and set the stage for future employment tensions.

Job interviews are also confronting for most autistic adults. They may come across as if they were applying for the CEO position, or, at the other extreme, as if they were underselling themselves. Employers may have no indication of the possible gem in front of them, whose weakest point may be poor interview skills. In a competitive market, a charismatic worker is more likely to be employed and promoted than a shy, competent, focused perfectionist who would be a real asset to the company.

A patchy resume or employment history is viewed unfavourably and may require explanation to prospective employers during interviews. This question is difficult for autistic adults to answer, as they don't clearly understand the dynamics themselves.

For adults, finding and keeping a suitable workplace is harder. A job might be perfect until a new boss takes over, or an autistic adult is relocated from a private workroom to a public office space, where they feel exposed. Because most workplaces are constantly evolving, this poses difficulty for anyone on the spectrum. They seek ways to cope, but much of this involves pushing their nerves to breaking point.

This is one reason many autistic people are diagnosed with depression. This is understandable after experiencing failed relationships, numerous job changes and upheaval in living arrangements, but it is often misleading. Depression may be a secondary issue in response to the frustration of struggling with autism.

If they could just tweak life a little in their favour, they could cope and hang on in an ever-changing world. A world that is too fast, too furious and too demanding! Then the vulnerability and anxiety that permeate their days and haunt their nights might be alleviated. For they also have a strong desire to achieve and to provide stability for those who depend on them.

The number of people in their lives is often carefully, if unconsciously, limited so they can survive in a world that pushes and pulls them at every turn. Each new solution to their internal dilemma, be it a new career or a relocation, is presented with intelligence, eloquence, and a compelling argument. An argument that will be debated and repeated until their point is conceded and the listener expresses understanding. Never mind that the current job or situation was previously touted as the answer to all problems; the new idea takes root. Their hope rises; family and friends can't help but be swept along on the tide of their buoyant mood. Maybe this time it will take. After all, their distress in the present circumstances is evident.

The people closest to them go with the flow, often failing to recognise the trend for what it is: anxiety-driven discomfort that is hot-wired into their brain function. It's very hard for even the most loving partner or parent to see the autistic person's difficulties as internal. This is because it's hard to find more loving, supportive and trustworthy people on the planet. They bring the added bonus of making a loved one feel needed, and they are needed, often with a desperation that discomforts the other person.

Those close to autistic people in this situation are often drawn into helping them achieve the position or change they want, persuaded by their explanation of the problem. The desire to help often leads the support person to bend and stretch to fit the autistic person. Because the autistic person presents their position and thoughts in such a compelling way to others, their argument appears all the more rational and reasonable. Whatever problem an autistic person has is accepted at face value by their support person. Those closest to the autistic person will then defend them against all comers, never realising that they are feeding the constant striving to change an external world rather than an internal one.

An autism diagnosis, however, opens the door to understanding. It may also bring relief. A sense of freedom often follows when the autistic person realises they are okay, have a future, and, most of all, now have choices. They can choose the environment that suits them, rather than face the constant demands to fit the job description. They may find a quiet corner at their workplace, perhaps a small office where the boss recognises their need for solitude and quiet and simply 'lets them get on with it'.

They might also decide to work from home, where they can control their hours, conditions, and even the clients they accept. Maybe they can free a partner to 'go forth and conquer' in their own employment and focus on being a parent. The options are endless and as varied as the individual. They can embrace the fact that they work best alone.

Hopefully, somewhere along the way, employers, higher education institutions, and the community will come to understand autistic people. Such understanding could dissolve the 'lazy, rude, indifferent, unmotivated' categories that autistic people currently inhabit. It would also make allowances in workplaces, communities and homes, enabling autistic people to become fully functioning, contributing members. of society.

I can't find my son!

Back in my hometown after leaving Adam and leaving Queensland, I made an offer on the worst house in the best street, and it was accepted. The colour scheme inside was appalling, and the shower leaked, but the layout was practical.

I brought in the painters. Gerard dismantled the leaking bathroom, and a friend relined it cheaply.

We had a home.

With five-year-old Bronson on access with Adam, I attempted to reintroduce myself to a social life. I arranged to go to the movies with a friend and Gerard. I thought I would relax, but soon discovered how hard it was. I didn't want to drive at night, and it was a long drive home from the movies.

I impressed on my thoughtful, malleable son that I needed him to drive, there and back home. Gerard had his full license and was a wonderful, calm driver, willing to drive anywhere. I hadn't been out for ages and had lost a lot of confidence.

My friend Lyn was coming with Gerard and me in my car. We met up with a carload of people who were Lyn's friends at the movie theatre.

The movie was great, the night was great, and then it was time to go home. When we came out of the movies, it was pitch black. I had been in another world for the past few hours and was disoriented by the darkness. I struggled to get my bearings. We all left to go to the cars. We didn't all get there.

I saw Gerard, my short-sighted son, come down the stairs into the parking lot, but when I arrived at the car, he wasn't there. I was mystified. I had seen him head across the car park.

I waited near the car. The minutes ticked by. I couldn't see Gerard anywhere. He had a great deal of patience with me, and I couldn't imagine what happened.

On a casual night out at the movies, only thirty kilometres from home, my panic reflex kicked in. I decided that some unseen force had taken him. The same unseen force pushed me over the edge between rationality and insanity. It was a rough ride, the destination as inevitable as night following day.

Every parent knows the sinking, ghastly feeling that assails you when you think that your child has gone missing. Some parents phone hospitals, some arrange funerals in their minds. As children, when my brother and I arrived home late, my mother would invariably say, 'We were just on our way to ring the Police!' My mother was the spokesperson for We. They had apparently been from anxiety to anger and back again several times without taking the car out of the garage.

I wandered the whole car park, moaning and wailing like a professional mourner, until there were no cars left. Lyn, a tall, cool blonde, was confused by my abandonment of the professional nurse in favour of the guise of a madwoman. She had never seen me like this, and after a brief attempt to rein me in, realised I was driving this train wreck, and nothing was going to stop me. My distress finally caught the security guard's attention with my plaintive, 'I can't find my son.' A lean man with a compassionate face, he saw at once the seriousness of the situation, or more likely was perplexed by such raw emotion, and promptly phoned the Police.

A burly officer with a thick blonde moustache attended the call and proceeded to sort out the dilemma. In true investigative style he began to question me.

'What is wrong, Madam?'

'I can't find my son.'

'How old is your son, Madam?'

'Seventeen.'

'And how tall is he?' At this particular point, a very small light came on in my brain. I ignored it and went for broke. I became a little vague.

'Oh, he's around 6 feet, I guess.'

'You mean to tell me that you have called me out to look for a seventeen-year-old boy who is about 6 feet tall! What do you expect me to do?' No sympathy here.

'Well,' said I, annoyed more by his attitude than the realities at this point, 'Well, pardon me, officer, I haven't been watching the news, I didn't realise that people of a certain age and size were exempt from being attacked, cut up in pieces and thrown over the fence. I don't know what you should do, I'm sure, I am his mother. I'm supposed to panic, and I am panicking. You must have gone to Police school to learn what to do in this kind of situation.'

At that, the officer got an unusual glint in his eye. I wondered if they had a code for 'I've got a live one'. Any minute now, he would put out an all-points bulletin nutcase alert. He must have decided to take valour over discretion. Smarter than me.

'Well, I can't do anything here; we'll have to go to the station.'

Not knowing how to leave well enough alone, I ploughed on, digging my own grave deeper by the minute.

'You mean to tell me that every 12-year-old on the North Shore has a mobile phone and the Government can't even supply the police force with walkie-talkie thingys?' An attempt to confound him with technical jargon failed as I forgot what to call them. He judiciously ignored this remark and told me to follow him to the station.

What followed can only be described as a high-speed police chase with all the road rules ignored. The only difference was that in this case, the suspect was trying to keep up with the Police. After weaving around in lanes all over Charlestown, we arrived at a squat dark building with one small flickering light vainly trying to dispel the darkness.

At this stage, all pretence at manners eluded the officer, and he disappeared into the building, leaving me in the parking lot. I was obviously at the back of the station, and I was furious. Emboldened by my new sense of injustice, I called out at the first available doorway, 'Am I supposed to follow you, or have you gone to the John?' This brave, rather loud statement was not met with silence but by the guffaws of his fellow officers who sensed some free entertainment. The red-faced officer returned to the parking lot to show me in.

When I arrived in the interview room, the place was packed with smiling policemen. The reluctance the sneering moustachioed officer had towards dealing with me had been replaced with a sincere desire to help me on my way with all possible speed.

We had met Lyn's friends at the movies. She told the officer, and he phoned them. Of course, they had all arrived home by this time, along with Gerard, and had even caught a little sleep. I couldn't believe that Gerard had immediately got a ride home with the others without looking for me or finding the car.

Common sense told me I might owe the officer an apology. Common sense did not prevail. Falsely assuming that things couldn't get any worse, the officer decided to show his magnanimous nature and invited me for 'coffee sometime'. This innocuous suggestion I refused out of hand. I was strangely reluctant to let go of the role of the wronged and misunderstood citizen. I was not to be placated. I very politely informed him just what he could do with his coffee.

I then decided on a suitably dramatic exit, thanked the officers, expressed concern for the rest of the night's entertainment and their imminent danger of boredom, wished them well, headed towards the dark doorway that appeared to be the exit, said goodnight, and walked straight into the cells.

'Shit!' I said.

A man called Ray

In my travels around our neighbourhood, I visited Ray, our neighbourhood eccentric. On one visit, Ray wanted to tell me that he had been kept awake at night with my security lights going off and lighting half the neighbourhood every time Diane's cat walked past.

Colourful obscenities peppered his speech. If I interrupted him, he would say, 'Will you ever shut up, you bitch, I am trying to talk to you!'

When I first arrived on the street, Ray wandered over to help out, something the big-hearted man did that my Christian neighbours did not do. He was astonished that I was furiously yanking out all the Venetian blinds in my new home.

'What the bloody hell are ya doin' that for?' he asked.

I told him the story of my childhood wrangling with venetian blinds. A story that featured my mother and my brother's dog, Snoopy.

Mum had a compulsion for cleaning everything within an inch of its life. These torturous cleaning processes at our house involved the windows. To be fair, they actually featured the windows, as they were most readily visible to all. Her usual method of masochism prevailed, and she insisted on each window having a full set of venetian blinds, sheer drapes and then heavy drapes. These were all religiously positioned by her at precise times of the day and night.

The cleaning of the whole lot was another matter entirely. The Venetians had to be removed by the tallest and most technical child, that being my father. Then they were hung from the clothesline, where it was my job to scrub every inch of them. To add to my torment, Snoopy, my brother's dog, was left tied to the clothesline to add further nuisance to the task.

The blasted dog raced around my feet and the clothesline until I invariably fell in the mud with my legs tangled in chains. This was high adventure for Snoopy, but it caused great wrath and resentment in me. No matter how pathetically I protested about his presence, Snoopy stayed chained to the clothesline.

When I related the story, Ray chortled an emphysemic laugh and helped me tear down the blinds and shove them in the whizz bin.

Gerard was seventeen. He and Ray hit it off immediately.

Gerard, who valued authenticity above all other virtues, found in Ray the epitome of charitable kindness.

I overheard Ray telling Gerard about a churchwoman who annoyed him by putting religious flyers in his letterbox and banging on about religion. 'Silly cow won't let up,' he told Gerard. 'So I told her to kiss my arse, but to wash her face first.'

Gerard repeated this story to all his friends with great enjoyment. Gerard tolerated personal intrusions, unwanted advice and preachy people with deference, although anyone who could see through his narrow-eyed gaze would know that he had found them wanting. Bronson, cut from a different cloth, answered the phone to one do-gooder with, 'Do you never shut up?' This technique was greatly admired by Gerard, and when the woman in question complained to him about his brother's behaviour, Gerard said,

'The kid is prone to tell the truth.'

Despite his language, he was the gentlest and most caring man, known for watering gardens, caring for pets, carrying groceries, and helping anyone.

Before I arrived in the area, Ray had been helping a neighbour, whose body was ravaged by cancer, to load his things to take to the retirement village. The local pastor arrived to collect the cheque for the retirement home. With his ragged appearance and perpetual fag hanging out of his mouth, Ray was immediately judged and questioned by the pastor. 'Don't worry, mate,' said Ray. 'I'm not thievin', I'm just helpin' the old guy out.'

This straightforward speech shocked the impeccably dressed pastor who had offered no assistance to the old man. It was just as well that Ray didn't get around to his usual language antics and say something that the poor pastor could never repeat to a living soul.

Ray had no time for 'religious types of any flavour.' If there is such a place as heaven, Ray will be shocked to find himself in a heaven he could not have imagined after living in a world with no God of love he could perceive.

I often visited Ray for a cuppa. When I arrived, I was greeted with, 'Go 'round the back, ya silly bitch, ya can't get in the front door.' We enjoyed a chat with only the occasional, 'Will you for Christ's sake, shut up.'

One day, the phone rang, and Ray greeted the caller with, 'How are you, ya sexual maniac?' This was apparently a devoted and favourite nephew enquiring after his health because he had undergone recent exhaustive medical tests for lung cancer.

'Oh no mate, I'm fucked,' he said. 'No, seriously, I'm dying, mate, yeah, got the cancer every which way 'til Sunday. No, I can't have the chemotherapy or the radiotherapy because of the open-heart surgery, but I won't be hitting the downhill slope until November. Don't let it worry you, mate, I will be around for a while yet, Christ doesn't want me, and the Devil is booked solid.'

After this cheerful exchange, he sat down and resumed his chat with me without losing a single thread of our conversation, quite possibly leaving a devastated nephew on the end of the phone line. Or perhaps the nephew knew this marvellous man and his incredible attitude to life well.

I sometimes gave Ray a lift into town or picked him up. One day, I had Bronson in the car.

'Christ Almighty girl, your driving will get me killed,' he said as I avoided another car leaving the grocery shop's car park.

'What do you care,' I said, 'you're dying anyway.'

Ray roared with laughter, while Bronson was shocked and appalled until he became accustomed to the banter between us and to Ray's marvellous attitude to life and death.

On another visit, I told Ray about my escapades with vandals, thieves and cops. I told him I had pressured the cops to do something. When I left, Ray sent his fond regards to Bronson, whom he regarded as a 'beaut little guy with lovely manners.' Ray told me to tell Bronson to come to him any time he was worried. One of the worst bullies lived opposite Ray. Ray started looking out for Bronson.

After a week or so, Ray rang me with his usual 'getting straight to the point' attitude.

'What 'ave you been up to ya bloody bitch? There hasn't been a kid in the street for the last week. Only a few really little tikes who seem really confused that they have the street to themselves and are making the most of it without the big bullies messin' with 'em and the main culprit hasn't come out of the back yard kickin' a football, and I never seen that kid look at a football before!'

Waterloo

As soon as we arrived in town, I started casual work with a nursing agency doing community nursing. I often had ten patients in a day; showering, dressing, washing, cooking, feeding pets, giving insulin injections, medications and treatments. I didn't work many days a week, but worked long hours. I typically arrived at my first patient by six in the morning, heading home for a break around two thirty in the afternoon to put on a load of washing and have lunch. I started back at three-thirty, often finishing the day well after nine.

I contracted Glandular Fever. Blood tests revealed that I had suffered from several major viruses previously. Long months later, after failing to respond and still suffering heavy flu-like symptoms, I was diagnosed with Chronic Fatigue Syndrome or ME.

I didn't have much energy to mourn the loss of my life.

With the flu, a few days of misery seem like a lifetime. With Chronic Fatigue, the flu symptoms last for days and nights for years. No anecdotal medical "evidence" of getting over it has any feel of reality. I felt like I was dying. Just surviving to be around for my boys was the limit of my daily struggle.

When I slowly began to recover, I looked at the house and was overwhelmed. I divided my life into bite-sized pieces and began to tackle the house, inch by inch. I worked out on the calculator how long it would take to get the house sorted if I tidied and cleaned one metre at a time and got started. Some days I could only do a few minutes at a time, and others an hour or two. I would lie down and then get up and get going again.

I scraped, scrubbed, puffed and sweated. I began to see possibilities in every corner. I was ruthless in sorting through the accumulated belongings and sent much to the Salvation Army. I never wanted to drown under clutter ever again. Some advances were hit and miss. I would shift the furniture and then want it to go somewhere else.

Opening the linen cupboard one day, I was hit with the smell of damp carpet. The shower had leaked into the cupboard. We needed to remove and replace the shower.

I got my tools out and started removing the bathroom tiles.

Gerard heard the noise and came to see what I was doing.

'Mum, you're wrecking every tile and making holes in the wall.'

I sighed. Sat on the edge of the bath. 'I know.'

Gerard took over, and with the same tool, gently prised every bathroom tile from the wall, leaving no holes, no noise, and no impatience.

Ramius – the thoroughbred moron

Pets are often extremely good therapy for children with autism or neurodivergence because the child doesn't have to interpret the social implications of their interaction with them.

The first pet to join the family was a part Persian moggy whose colouring could best be described as splotchy. Orange, brown and white, she brought delight into our lives and soon earned the name of Rug, due to her ability to settle herself into a comfortable spot and imitate a rug.

Her relaxed attitude may have had something to do with the fact that Gerard had turned eighteen and both he and the cat were partial to a drop of Southern Comfort.

The next kitten was a funny little thing with a crooked leg.

'Trust you, Mum,' said Gerard, 'to bring home a kitten with a dud leg.'

I hadn't even noticed.

Gerard bought a Russian Blue kitten and named it Ramius. Ramius was an elegant, condescending moggy that Gerard often referred to as a thoroughbred moron. Ramius was not up to the usual challenges of felineness. Not for him the fighting and playfulness of the other kittens. The only scampering he attempted was when loud noises scared the crap out of him, and he fled.

Under siege

Adam's anger continued after we moved back to my hometown. He began following me, which is more commonly called stalking. He hid behind a tree across the road until the owner of the property got sick of it and chopped the tree down. I didn't know I was being stalked until I was told about the tree, and several of Gerard's friends said they had seen Adam here, or there.

While the boys and I were staying with my mother, Adam came around to her house. He bashed on the front door, yelling for Gerard to come out 'like a man.'

Gerard was out with mates. Mum was visiting a friend. I was alone with Bronson and afraid. Adam was yelling, and he showed no sign of slowing down or leaving. I went to the back room of the house and shut myself in with three-year-old Bronson, who was confused.

Adam kept hurling abuse, directed at Gerard. He didn't seem to work out that Gerard wasn't there. If Gerard had been there, he would have acted swiftly and phoned the police and several of his friends. He wouldn't have cowered in a back room like me.

If Mum had been there, she would have opened the door to confront Adam, which would have given Adam the opportunity to push his way inside, something he had done with our Toowoomba church pastor and others. I sometimes wish Mum had been there because she had trouble seeing past Adam's public persona of calm politeness.

Bronson went to sleep.

Adam grew louder. It was clear he wasn't just going to leave. Keeping low, I crawled to the kitchen, where I felt exposed. I phoned 000 and shivered behind Mum's kitchen bench. Adam was only metres away at the front door, with full view of the lounge and kitchen. He kept yelling for Gerard to 'come out and be a man.'

After hearing my breathless summary of the situation and gaining the address, the police informed me that they were already on their way. Someone else had heard and reported it.

The police arrived, and a tense standoff ensued. I stayed inside as two policemen stood on the verge and carried on a conversation with Adam, who was not intimidated by their presence and began to include them in the rant, veering seamlessly into the victim mode of a deprived father. 'You cop's don't understand. Always on the woman's side. A man has a right to see his son!' Adam's focus had quickly shifted from abusing Gerard.

The officers reasoned.

Adam ranted.

The cops finally prevailed, and Adam stormed off, promising legal carnage and retribution.

Mum arrived home, shocked to see the police in her front yard. She had never seen police attend any type of neighbourhood or family drama.

I came out and spoke to the officers. 'Why didn't you come up to the door to talk to him?' I asked. 'I was so afraid.'

'We're not allowed on the property. We can't use force. We had to persuade him to leave.'

'Good grief,' I said, 'this is why women are reluctant to phone the police. You don't have any greater power than we women do.'

'We have to advise you to get an AVO with the magistrate.'

'Sure,' I said, 'another thing to enrage Adam and make me less safe. Sure.'

They took some time explaining. Apparently, 99% of men stop the behaviour. It wasn't until they said, 'an AVO gives us the power to arrest and remove…' that I agreed. The magistrate immediately granted the AVO I requested. The police report probably helped.

The next time that Adam called for access, my brother was visiting from WA. He had a black belt in karate and had attended exhibitions in Japan, but unlike Adam, his calm gentility never wavered.

Gerard walked out and stood near Adam. 'I hear you had something to say to me.'

Adam demurred.

Wordlessly, with just a familiar tweak of his mouth, my brother ushered Bronson forward.

Handover was different that day.

Gerard later told me how much these interactions affected him.

'Were you afraid?' I asked.

'Of course, Mum. The man's a psychopath.'

I was at the local courthouse one hot Tuesday in the middle of an Australian heat wave. There, once more, for an AVO because as soon as one order expired, Adam started stalking me again.

At the hearings, Adam invariably sought an adjournment. By about the third time there, I was getting a little braver. After all, there were police officers everywhere. The young female solicitors from the community Family Law service who represented women in family violence situations were firm, professional and unflinching. With their hair coiled tightly, they wore sharp suits and had sharp words to match. I just had to turn up and let them lead.

However, on this day I was informed that none of these fierce girls was available and I would have to have whoever was available, which might mean getting someone unfamiliar with family violence.

I waited. And waited.

My new legal aid solicitor finally arrived in a fluster. She was a plump middle-aged woman in a pleated skirt and a pastel sweater. After expressing relief at finding me, she asked me to point out my ex-husband. Her eyes glazed over. She saw this tall, marvellous specimen with his shiny shoes and diffident manner. She sighed softly and said, 'Ha. You won't win. You won't get anything against THAT MAN. Trust me.'

She promptly wandered off to gather "something", disappearing in the crowd.

I decided I would represent myself. How could I expect anything from that woman?

I found the main office. 'Um,' I said to the lady at the desk, 'is it okay for someone to represent themselves?'

'Yes, certainly,' she said, 'the men often do. We haven't had a woman ask, but why not?' She smiled. I was encouraged. I told her that my legal aid solicitor looked at my ex-husband as if he were George Clooney. She made a choking sound, and several other staff members poked their heads up from their tasks.

'Do you know what to say?' she asked.

'No,' I said, 'I never do. But I figure all I have to do is tell the truth and be humble.'

'That'll do it,' she said, 'rarer than you might think.'

I walked into the courtroom and was surprised to find the room packed. I had to walk to the front, past Adam, who was in deep conversation with a suited man I didn't know.

The next case was announced. A beautiful thin woman with flowing blonde hair stood. She was sobbing pitifully with a pale girl clinging to her skirts. Bruises were evident on the woman. The defendant, her handcuffed ex-partner, was escorted by two burly policemen into the court. He was placed in the dock where he sat scruffy and defiant. I was shocked. I wasn't expecting this malarkey.

Through her solicitor, the tearful woman asked for an AVO and for police officers to be present when her violent ex came to the flat to collect his belongings.

Clearly unimpressed, the magistrate frowned. 'The police have better things to do than help collect belongings when people can't work out their own lives.'

This caused more sobbing from the frail creature. It also had the effect on the moron in the dock to feel emboldened to assume that he was now the wronged party, and he began to babble to the magistrate.

The magistrate turned to him. 'Excuse me, Mr G! You are the one in the dock in handcuffs here, and you are going back downstairs to the cells shortly. Don't get any ideas about yourself!'

The magistrate swiftly determined that the woman could organise one of her family members to be present when the moron came to collect his things. The gavel banged. The policemen collected the moron.

I swallowed—hard. Adam and I were up next on the roster. This magistrate was going to eat me. He had berated a fragile waif of a woman with a clinging child, and her criminal ex. There I was with the gall to eschew legal representation. How could I explain my decision? Tell the magistrate I felt I didn't stand a chance with a legal aid solicitor who showed signs of fancying my ex-husband?

The clerk called our case. Matter No#. Dixon vs Dixon. The suited man beside Adam stood, clearly a solicitor. I stood where the clerk indicated. The magistrate inclined his head in recognition of Adam's solicitor and then asked if I was representing myself.

'Yes, Your Honour.'

He nodded. Thankfully, he did not question my sanity, which was truly soothing as I was doing enough of that myself.

Adam's solicitor began. 'Mr Dixon requests that there be an

adjournment of three weeks, your honour.'

The magistrate turned to me. 'Do you wish to oppose this, Mrs Dixon?' he politely enquired.

'Well, your honour, does Mr Dixon have the right to postpone the hearing?' I politely enquired.

'Yes, he does, Mrs Dixon.'

'Well then, Your Honour, I see no point in objecting.'

The gavel banged. The appointment book was sought. Hearing set down for the blah blah.

I walked out on air.

After a few more adjournments, despite bringing a solicitor, Adam couldn't resist standing up and interjecting loudly.

'I wish to protest that MY wife gets to speak and MY voice is not heard. It is grossly unfair.'

The magistrate rewarded this belligerence with, 'Mr Dixon. You have paid good money for someone else to represent you. Sit down and be quiet.'

The gavel was banged in my favour with very few words from me and the absence of any legal strategy whatever.

Adam accused me of using "your clever mouth" to impress the judge, an accusation he often levelled at me. I merely smiled and thought, 'Yes, I kept it shut.'

Tuesdays

Tuesday was the day when applications for apprehended violence orders were heard at the local court.

Gerard came with me the first time I went to court for an AVO. He walked with me into the waiting room filled with other women seeking AVOs.

There was a collective gasp in the room by the battered wives at the sight of a large male.

Gerard knew instantly. Felt it like a heartbeat, a pulse. He put a large hand on my shoulder. 'I'm just here for my mother.'

He sighed, a chest heave.

'I'm sorry,' he said, 'I'm sorry on behalf of all men. The men who have done this to you. Filled you with fear. I'm just here for my mother, but I'll wait outside. I don't want to discomfort you.'

'Stay,' they said, 'please stay,' they said, wishing for sons like Gerard. Men like Gerard.

Gerard studied law at university. Some of his classmates remarked on his size and masculinity and said, 'I guess you'll make a pile of money making sure men get everything in divorces.'

'I'm only going to represent single mothers,' Gerard said.

Adam adjourned every hearing, thinking to discomfort me, but I actually began to enjoy these outings to the court.

I came dressed for the part. I wore a fitted navy suit that I had made, a white silk cowl-neck blouse, navy stockings and high heels. I wore make-up and had my hair up. I carried a black briefcase that anyone would have been surprised to discover held my shopping list.

I arrived early. I walked past the crowd waiting outside with their peasant tops, checked flannelette shirts and thongs and went inside to the toilets. I was delighted to hear someone say, 'The solicitors have started to arrive.'

Safely seated on the court benches outside, waiting to be called, I engaged in one of my favourite pastimes of people watching. I was amazed when one mother lifted her child up by the arm and thoroughly whacked its bum in full view of several policemen, the court officers and the rest of us who would soon be in the gallery.

By the fourth time, I was getting a bit bored, so I started to enter conversations with complete strangers. I found that sitting at court brought out the strange propensity for people to talk to themselves, and I have always assumed that this was an invitation for anyone present to join in.

One day, I was next to a well-dressed, dark-haired man of Mediterranean descent who kept repeating to himself, 'I don't know why I'm here?'

At first, I answered him silently in my head with the thought, 'Hello, it is Tuesday, the day put aside for domestic violence or the occasional murder—and those boys are usually wearing handcuffs and have personal escorts.'

After he repeated this several times, I felt compelled to explain life to him. I started innocently enough—a sign my friends would have recognised as trouble but not him, 'So, you don't understand?'

This seemingly sympathetic remark loosened his tongue considerably. He didn't seem to notice that he was surrounded by quite a few other people, engaged in fear, boredom, and apprehensive chain-smoking, and there was a woman on the other side of me who was enthusiastically wailing her way through a large box of tissues that her friend held helplessly in front of her.

'I thought we were happy, I thought we had a great marriage, twenty years together, and I never saw it coming. Why didn't I see this coming?' moaned the unfortunate, deserted man.

I stepped it up a notch.

'Well, darling, that's because you are a man.' I now had his full attention. And that of several others I suspected. I swear I don't set out to do this. It just happens. His eyes now beseeched me for answers. I knew I was wasting my time, but I thought, what the hell, I'm bored.

I continued, 'Well, this is how it goes, a woman gets up in the morning and thinks about the relationship, she has breakfast and thinks about the relationship, she takes the kids to school and thinks about the relationship, she has coffee with friends and thinks about the relationship, she goes to work and thinks about the relationship and then she comes home, gets tea, washes the dishes watches a little television and she is still thinking about the relationship.'

I paused, embarrassed to find all eyes on me. The woman who had been copiously going through the Kleenex had stopped crying and was staring at me, open-mouthed. Her friend started to giggle.

'But you,' I continued, 'get up and have breakfast and think about breakfast, you go to work and think about work, you have a few beers with your mates and think about your mates, you come home and read the newspaper and think about the newspaper, you watch TV and think about the TV program—your wife has had twenty years up on you of thinking about this and working it out and it's over sweetheart!'

And about his time, the timid chuckles of the Kleenex lady had joined with the snorts from her friend, and as the newly informed man went back to his confused reverie, we women had a wonderful chat, and the tissues were handed around to all for laughter instead.

Defamation

The next time I saw Adam, he told me that he had engaged a solicitor and would be suing me for defamation. I would soon receive a letter. His father had 'heard rumours' and was affronted by the family name being dragged through the mud.

'I guess that means that your father has forgotten the time he was drunk and stormed down the main street in his underpants with a rifle looking for the local police sergeant. I guess he has forgotten the years of family abuse, chasing his own children with a rifle and peppering the trees at the local park with bullets as you four kids hid behind trees. He'll make an excellent witness.'

Adam flushed. 'I … I have heard stuff too.'

'Oh, good luck with that.' How little Adam knew. How little he knew how effectively he had silenced me. How afraid I was to reveal anything to friend or foe.

'By the way, you don't have to worry about your family name because I have legally returned to my maiden name. Taking the name of a man worthy of respect. Please remember that in the future.'

Bronson's Hero

Gerard was his brother's first hero.

After his stepfather had been shipwrecked from the marriage, Gerard continued to step up, usually in response to the noise level created by Bronson.

Gerard's consistent gentleness therapy, while not actually brushing off on Bronson, did serve to forge a beautiful bond. Gerard could achieve what no one else could. This led to a measure of frustration on my part and a certain amount of self-righteousness on his. I was too desperate for peace and answers to let this get in the way of something that was working.

When Bronson was four, screaming loudly, afraid he would drown in an inch of bath water, Gerard was there to reassure him and show him how to take a shower. When Bronson threw a tantrum, kicking and screaming, Gerard got right down there with him and threw a better one before quietly saying, 'Now, that didn't do any good, did it?' That was the end of the tantrum. Whether this was because Bronson was in awe of a superior tantrum or he had actually learned something, I cannot say. I do know that whenever Bronson was in the midst of chaos, his brother's outstretched hand usually brought the drama to an end. Gerard provided his brother with stability, wisdom, love, and the gentleness that therapy and the lessons he learned and inherited from his grandfather, Max, brought him. His explanations and admonitions were short and clear.

Gerard let Bronson invade his sacred teenage domain and pull all the books from his bookshelf. He made him walk further when he was whining and tired, made him eat different foods, and made him throw up his bottle.

Always patient, he forced Bronson to share his toys, toys that Gerard didn't really want to, just to teach a lesson about sharing. One Christmas, he bought Bronson a lawnmower that made a shocking racket so Bronson could follow him around the yard while he was mowing. He made Bronson wash up every day, even when Bronson declared this to be child abuse.

One of the best things Gerard ever did was to sit and watch the Disney animated movie version of "The Hunchback of Notre Dame" with Bronson and talk to him about "what makes a monster and what makes a man".

In the manner of all big brothers, he teased him and rumbled him; called him names like "tosser" and "wally", woke him up in the middle of the night when Bronson was talking in his sleep to have silly conversations with him, with Bronson declaring that 'they didn't have enough penguins to win the war.' He dealt with the double standard of not allowing Bronson to swear because he 'wasn't old enough and couldn't do it right.' Even though he was eighteen, he ran around the neighbourhood with water pistols at the ready until both he and Bronson were drenched and laughing.

When Bronson was two, Gerard sat him on the swing outside, telling him to stop his cranky-boy routine of yowling and giving people headaches.

Sometimes he united with Bronson in 'rebellion against the mother.' At other times, he said, 'Be good to her, she's my mother too, you know.' When he was only about sixteen, I asked Gerard what the best thing I had ever done for him was. He said, 'Giving me Bronson, because now I know I will be a good father.'

Solemn and wonderful words from a boy who didn't know what it was to have a father.

Gerard didn't want his brother to ever get mixed up about what made a monster and what made a man. They watched Disney movies together despite the fourteen-year difference. I had enough Disney DVDs to start my own movie theatre. I'm not sure how or when, but The Hunchback of Notre Dame became a favourite for the brothers. I would hear the subtle murmur of Gerard's voice as he asked his small brother questions throughout the movie. 'Which one is the monster and which one is the man?' Gerard asked, keeping his own opinions and experiences of men and monsters to himself.

'I dunno. Everyone is treating poor Quasimodo as if he's the monster because his body is twisted,' said Bronson, writhing his hands to demonstrate, 'but he's kind to small creatures, and he's only angry when he protects Esmeralda, the gypsy girl, who's bullied and spat on and stuff.'

'Does having a twisted body make a man a monster, then?'

'No, it makes him picked on and made to do stuff.'

'What about Captain Phoebus? Was he a good man or a bad man?'

'He took a bit of time to make up his mind, but he got there in the end. So he's good.'

'What about Frollo? The Judge with the fine clothes and the power? The one who prays for justice?'

'He's a right bastard,' said Bronson.

'You reckon he's the monster then?'

'Yep, fine prayers, fancy words and 'spensive clothes don't make him a man. Suits and prayers – tell ya nothin'.'

'You think you'll remember then? What makes a monster and what makes a man?'

'Yep, won't fool me with that stuff. I like that Esmeralda,' said small brother.

'She's not half bad in the flesh either,' said Gerard, perhaps remembering other movies with Demi Moore.

'Huh?'

'Never mind.'

A wedding

'Mum needs to be near a toilet all the time,' announced Bronson to the air hostess.

I moaned. It was our first plane trip. Bronson was nine. We were travelling from Sydney to Brisbane for Gerard's wedding. While we were on the plane, Bronson was more interested in informing everyone of my medical problems than enjoying the flight.

'She's had an operation, and now she needs to *go* a lot. All the time, actually. It's a bloody nuisance,' he confided loudly to the hostess. She smothered a smile. I leaned back in the chair, hoping this was not a sign of things to come.

The wedding was going to be held at the retirement village where Gerard's great-grandmother, Ruby, was a resident. It was also her 100th birthday, so relatives had come from far and wide. Essentially, this was a family reunion for the large clan of Gerard's relatives. Plus my mother, Bronson and I.

We were staying for a week. Mum stayed with an old friend. I hardly saw her. Bronson and I were staying with my Auntie Di.

Bronson's sense of adventure deserted him because he had traded aeroplanes, instruments and gadgets for people—strangers. There was only one person Bronson would endure this for, his beloved brother.

Gerard's father, Guy, was attending with his wife, Dana and their three children. This was a reunion for Guy with his firstborn son after 18 years. Gerard met Guy's children, Gerard's half-brothers and his half-sister.

He introduced Bronson to them. 'These are my brothers and my sister,' said Gerard.

Damien, Guy's middle child, was yanking on Gerard's hand and dancing around, babbling loudly.

'Is *he* my brother too?' asked Bronson, eyeing Damien, his face awash with confusion.

'No, he's my brother,' answered Gerard.

'How come you have a brother that isn't my brother?'

'Because Damien and I have the same father, but different mothers,' Gerard said. 'Actually, these are my half-brothers, and Crystal is my half-sister.'

'Don't be stupid,' said Bronson. 'You can't have half people.'

'Gerard is your half-brother as well, Bronson,' added a well-meaning passerby.

'You're all stupid!' declared Bronson, dismissing the whole gathering as beyond help. He was insulted beyond belief. This big brother he had known and loved all his life was no half to him.

Bronson took an instant dislike to Damien, and the feeling was mutual. Damien had accepted his new big brother as both a hero and a friend. Bronson's nose was thoroughly out of joint. He looked at Damien as if he were a hyperactive terrorist.

'Why is he so loud?' asked Bronson, covering his ears.

'He doesn't know he's being loud because he can't hear,' someone said. 'He's deaf.'

'Well, why doesn't someone make him write things down? He *can* write, can't he?'

Thankfully, Bronson and Damien managed to avoid conflict. Mainly because Bronson withdrew and teamed up with a quiet boy who shared the same Pokémon obsession.

I had a great time reconnecting with Guy's brothers and sister. I had been an integral part of their lives before the divorce, and we fell back into an easy camaraderie. I was included in many family meals, but I spent most of my time with Bronson or my aunt.

Gerard and Liane were going to be married by Gerard's paternal grandfather, a pastor, the day after the birthday party for Gerard's great-grandmother, Ruby. Ruby had cared for me after our second son was born. She was a fabulous cook and an impressive matriarch, but to me she was a dear friend.

It was great to catch up with Guy's cousins. Nerida and I had trained together at the same hospital, and I had seen a lot of Guy's other cousins. We had enjoyed the beach, dinners and outings together. I was greeted with excitement, but not by all. Guy's parents were extremely polite; however, their discomfort was obvious to me, if not to others. They had been vocal in the championship of Guy, and I was very aware that they had been equally vocal about my shortcomings.

I was tacitly invited to the birthday celebrations, but didn't plan to attend. This plan went awry when Bronson followed his new friend into the party. I couldn't let Bronson roam loose among the honoured guests, so I legged it to the venue, possibly a little less formally dressed than some of those honoured guests. I was greeted with pursed lips and surprise by Guy's parents, but I was soon surrounded by friends, former high school teachers, my nursing mentor from the medical centre where I had worked, and all of Guy's relatives of my age. After all, we had all grown up in the same religion.

After the party ended, a wedding rehearsal was arranged. Bronson was required to attend, but I relaxed, put on shorts and a T-shirt, and settled in to spend time with my aunt. Bronson would be on his best behaviour around Gerard.

Unfortunately, my presence was requested. I was confused by this, as I wasn't part of the wedding party, even though I had teased Gerard that I should be his Best Woman, since none of his friends could attend.

With no time to change, I did as I was bidden and went to the chapel. Inappropriately dressed. Again.

Gerard's father and grandfather were in their element. Born charismatics and organisers, they waved their arms and issued instructions like zealous conquerors.

I was told to sit behind the piano.

I then realised why my presence had been requested. I was to be sidelined for the wedding.

The following day, I arrived at the chapel early, dressed appropriately for the wedding. My hair was coiled, my dress swirled, and my heart thundered.

Guy was at the front with Gerard as his son's best man. Guy's wife sat in the front row with their children. Bronson was as near to his brother as he dared in a suit and tie.

I stood at the back of the chapel, unsure, wrong-footed as the other guests entered and took their places. I looked over at the seats behind the piano where I was supposed to sit, but they were taken by sightseeing residents of the village.

The longer I stood there, the closer I came to tears. There were no ushers. And there was no place for me.

The music began. Guests quietened. Papers shuffled. No one noticed. I couldn't see my mother anywhere.

Gerard radiated happiness. He had fallen deeply and desperately in love with Liane, and even though he hated being the centre of attention, he relished his role as groom and husband-to-be on this day.

Gerard spied me standing at the back and smiled.

He left the front of the church and walked the long aisle towards me. He hooked my arm through his, led me to the front pew, then returned to his designated spot among the bridal party and waited for his bride.

The USA

Reconnecting with his father at his wedding encouraged both father and son to follow through with a visit to America, where Guy lived. Gerard was upset that Guy wouldn't pay for Liane to go as well, but he accepted and flew out to the USA. Gerard hoped to pay for Liane to join him. His father had promised to give him some work and pay him.

During this new relationship building, Guy began to realise how different they were. Gerard didn't enjoy the bountiful gift of going to Disneyland. He wasn't interested in going on any of the rides or seeing any of the sights, preferring to sit and watch proceedings from one of the Disneyland cafés.

Guy hired two Harley-Davidson motorcycles, and this pleased Gerard greatly. Gerard checked everything while Guy waited. Gerard prepared while Guy sighed.

They set off down a coastal road in California. Gerard took his time to enjoy the ride, and it wasn't long before Guy was out of sight. Gerard was lost and did the most reasonable thing. He saw two policemen and pulled in behind them.

The cops took one look at Gerard's bulk, his shaved head and goatee and rested their hands on their weapons. Their stance was obvious. There had been trouble with bikers. However, as soon as

Gerard spoke, they relaxed. 'You an Aussie mate?'

'Yeah, a bit obvious, right!' Gerard spent a congenial time chatting to the two officers and finally met up with Guy, who claimed to be worried out of his mind.

'Not five anymore, Dad,' said Gerard.

My father's rabbit

'I killed my father's rabbit and broke his heart,' I confided to Gerard as he put new brake pads on my front brakes.

We had been chatting about general things, and as soon as the words were out of my mouth, I wanted to take them back, desperately. When would I learn to choose the right moment? But then again, there never seemed to be a right moment for so many things I said, so I just sighed and hoped he hadn't heard.

'You did what?' he asked, putting down the tool he was holding. I looked over at his pet rabbit, Flopsy, the one with the permanently bent ear that scared the crap out of the neighbourhood cats. I'd been staring at Flopsy for five minutes with the warm sun on my back and floating back into the past.

'I killed my father's rabbit and broke his heart,' I repeated. I was sunk anyway. There was no taking it back now. Not with Gerard. I sighed. 'Dad had a pet rabbit named Benny that would jump up into his lap. It would run around the yard, never going far. And it would always come back to Dad. Dad built a terrific hutch for his rabbit, and when I was a kid, it was my job to put hessian bags over the hutch every night to keep it warm in winter. I got up one morning, and there was a huge fuss in the kitchen. My brother looked pale, and Mum was ranting and raving. She gave me a hard look when I came into the room, then pointed at me. "There's the culprit," she said accusingly. "It's her job to cover the hutch". The rest became a blur as I heard…frozen stiff…poor thing…didn't have a chance…never trust Linda with anything…" I ran out of the house like a criminal on the run. I went to hide behind the dunny only to find Dad there, weeping for Benny. I was crushed. I had never seen Dad shed a tear, and there he was sobbing for Benny. His heart was broken, and it was my fault. Benny had frozen to death, and it was my fault.'

Gerard looked gobsmacked. I waited for condemnation, hanging my head.

'For God's sake, Mum, how could you believe that rubbish! Have you ever told anyone this?'

'Of course not, silly, who confesses to killing their father's beloved bunny!'

Gerard grinned broadly. 'Silly little mother, rabbits come from England. They live *in the snow*. The bloody rabbit died in the night of natural causes and was stiff with rigor mortis.'

'So you don't put bags on Flopsy's hutch?'

'God no, hessian bags on a hutch wouldn't keep the cold out anyway. He has been outside through three winters! We come out in the morning, and he is happily nibbling grass with ice on his whiskers. Geez, poor silly mother.'

'So I don't need to knit Flopsy a jumper,' I said, fighting back tears.

Gerard came purposefully around the car and held me in his arms. 'You daft woman! You didn't kill your father's rabbit, and you never broke his heart.'

Good news and bad news

Gerard wandered up my driveway. It was getting dark, and I invited him in.

'Nah, Mum. I just came to tell you that Liane is pregnant. We're having a baby. I gotta get back.'

He showed no excitement even though he had longed to be a father. This confused me at the time, but when Gerard was given the autism diagnosis, it explained his mood. However, there were other things weighing heavily on him.

My mother, Gerard's grandmother, had fallen in her bathroom, tripping over the shower chair on the way to the toilet. She bravely soldiered on with fractured vertebrae, but one day she phoned for me to come to her unit. She needed me.

When I arrived, I saw a suitcase and knew what that meant. The pain had become too much. Mum had never willingly gone to the hospital. She'd had many visits there as emergencies, a spiral fracture to the leg, and urinary tract infections due to diabetes.

Gerard and Liane often took her to specialist appointments and visited her. But this time, she wanted the practical daughter, who would understand and support her submission and not fight against it.

She was admitted to Toronto Private Hospital, where pain therapy and rehabilitation began. Mum, who had never taken aspirin for pain, was fonder of the morphine than the rehabilitation.

'They make me go to the therapy place upstairs and do exercises,' she moaned to Bronson.

'That's awful,' said Bronson, 'What's wrong with people? They should just leave an old lady alone.'

'You're a sensible boy, Bronson,' Mum said, giving Gerard a stern warning look.

Gerard had not faced the reality that his 90-year-old Nan was facing the time when she could no longer live at home and needed to be in a nursing home.

My brother arrived from Perth and joined the Keep Nana at Home campaign, despite medical advice. The staff arranged an assessment. Mum had to walk, dress, eat and cook porridge. She held her head high as the assessment results were given to the family. Until one of the assessors who had overseen her cooking assessment walked in.

'Bother,' said Mum, 'I nearly burnt you with porridge. I'm done for, aren't I?

Mum suffered from dementia at the time, although Gerard and my brother resisted the diagnosis.

'She's fine when I'm there,' said my brother, a statement I had heard for decades as a registered nurse.

'She claimed to see giraffes in the rehab room. She argued with the staff that she was dead and didn't need them. She thought the cleaner was her doctor. One day, she was convinced that she was the Matron,' I said.

My brother gave me a superior look and argued politely with the staff when they tried to explain Mum's need to get sorted for nursing home admission. With Gerard on board the Keep Nana at Home train, my words were ignored.

One day, the ward sister expressed her frustration to me. 'We need papers signed, otherwise your mother will be transferred to any random nursing home at the end of her private hospital insurance cover. I don't know what to do with those two,' she said, referring to Gerard and my brother.

'I'm Mum's health guardian. She set this up with her solicitor. I'll sign them now.'

She brought the papers. I signed them, then informed the others that I had the legal right to do so and that Mum would be going to the nursing home connected to her current retirement village and not to some random place far away.

The family was not impressed. I was not included in family dinner gatherings.

Gerard sat with Mum and said, 'Nana. I'm your soldier, and I'm going to fight for you to stay in your unit.'

Mum eyed him as if he had lost his mind. 'I'm going to the nursing home. The one that Pa was in.'

'But Nan, if they cut your pain relief a bit, you'll be able to manage.'

Mum gave him a brutal stare and said firmly, 'Don't touch my morphine!'

Mum was transferred to the nursing home, where her confusion increased. She lost weight and motivation. She gripped my hand in a new way. 'Linda, getting old is horrible. I understand how Pa felt now.'

Gerard and Liane were desperate for Mum to live long enough to meet the new baby, but life had other plans. Mum died in my arms, after struggling to sit up for one last kiss on her cheek.

A daughter

'Mum, I need you.' Gerard's voice was strained. I checked the time. It was nearing midnight. 'Liane is having the baby, and she won't push.'

'Oh, dear.'

'Mum!'

'Yes, Gerard.'

'Can you come? I need you to come.'

'Liane will never forgive me. If I show up there, she'll…'

'I don't care. I need you.'

'How many years will I spend in the wilderness of estrangement over this,' I said, quietly gathering my purse and keys. 'How will I ever get into the hospital at this time of night, let alone walk onto a Maternity ward and into a labour suite?'

'You'll work it out, Mum. You always do. I need you. Never mind about Liane … Mum … Mum, why've you gone quiet?'

'I'm trying to pull my jeans on.'

'Then you're coming?'

'Did you ever doubt it?'

A sigh.

I still can't explain how I managed it. I walked through the doors of a hospital that I had never visited before, as if I owned the place. I strode across the foyer, nodded nonchalantly at a security guard as if I was a visiting dignitary, followed the signs and caught the lift to the Maternity Ward. I poked my head in several empty labour suites and walked into the room where Liane lay prostrate, and Gerard paced.

The maternity staff didn't seem to notice my arrival.

A blonde woman hovered at the business end of the delivery bed, taking a casual glance from the site of the prospective action and then at the belligerent patient. 'One more push,' she said. '

'You're bloody lying,' said Liane. 'I'm not listening to you again. One more push! One more push! You told me it was the last push hours ago.'

'Just one more push,' said the doctor, failing to realise that this statement had caused the mutiny in the first place.

Liane waved the gas mask around. 'And thish. Thish piece of shit,' she slurred, 'this does nothing. NOTHING!'

'It will if you keep it on.'

'Fuck it. I want another epidural. This one hasn't worked properly. It's only worked on half my body, and I want the other half fixed.'

'You can't have another epidural. Just one more push,' said the blonde woman reasonably. Her voice was soft and demure.

'Fuck you,' said Liane. 'You're fucking lying.' She threw her head back and mumbled about lying medicos.

'How far along is she?' I asked anyone who cared to answer. I hadn't worked out the hierarchy of the place, but I was beginning to understand why Gerard had phoned me.

'She's fully dilated,' said the quiet blonde, 'if she doesn't push the baby out, we're facing foetal distress.'

I was facing quite a bit of distress myself, but my reluctant daughter-in-law didn't blink an eye at the news. She probably hadn't heard the woman's soft voice.

Ignoring everyone, I lifted Liane's head and turned it towards me, and began to kiss her face.

'They're not lying, Liane. Your baby has to come out now. You have to push. You are going to save your baby's life.'

'Fuck me,' she said, then pushed with a roar, hurtling her newborn daughter into the cold, cruel world where mothers are lied to, and doctors fail to give adequate analgesia.

Gerard collapsed into my arms, then immediately accepted his new daughter, viewing her with the kind of wonder every woman wants to see.

I stayed to cut the cord. I took the first photos of Gerard holding the baby. My granddaughter.

Driving home, I wept. How long would it be before I was evicted from their lives again? It had become so habitual that Bronson had started to refer to the occurrence as 'being voted off the island'.

It was longer than usual. Liane needed a babysitter so she could return to work and fulfil her obligations under her maternity leave. As the only viable option, I was given the babysitting gig. I tried to hide how excited this made me.

When I babysat Daisy, her bright eyes followed me everywhere. Her tiny hand sneaked towards the computer cords, fingers twitching behind her back.

I was given a subtle hint that it would not be good form to do any household chores while I was babysitting, but I did anyway. I washed, dried and folded clothes, earning the side-eye of the mistress of the house, but she had more time to complete and no other viable (willing) option. Besides, I got bored.

I carried Daisy with me outside to pick lemons from the tree, to gurgle over Flopsy Bunny and lie on my stomach in the newly mown grass. I set her up in her highchair when I washed dishes, giving her plastic odds and ends to throw in the sudsy sink. I bathed her and diapered her, buying and using the miracle nappy cream that my friend Venessa had recommended when I had Bronson. I played silly games with Daisy. I lay on the floor and let her climb all over me. She giggled every time she saw me and reached for me when I was permitted entrance to the kingdom, wondering how long this halcyon period would last.

Liane completed her work requirement during her maternity leave and left work. I experienced a flutter of dread.

Gerard started cleaning the shed, an ominous sign that they were planning to move again, although I kept those thoughts to myself, afraid that bringing it into the open might upset the fine balance of our relationship. They had moved often, whenever a job didn't pan out for one or the other of them.

Gerard had a complicated system set up in the large garage. Huge barrels of a certain type of fish. Some sort of aquaponic arrangement where fish poo water runs through a conduit to grow lettuce. As usual, it was an ambitious system that Gerard had scientifically researched. It was, to quote Mother Earth News et al, "a sustainable, soil-less farming method that combines aquaculture (raising fish) with hydroponics (growing plants) in one integrated, recirculating ecosystem. Fish waste provides an organic nutrient source for the plants, and the plants act as a natural filter, cleaning the water for the fish."

When Bronson visited, he politely observed the system and admired the spindly lettuce he mistook for grass, the lawn kind.

The pipes were being dismantled. I never knew what happened to the fish. They were so small I had to pretend I could see them in the murky barrels.

I was in an agony of foreboding. I thought back to a few months before when Liane had left Gerard. She went to care for her mother after surgery, planning to stay for two weeks, but on the day of her planned return, she phoned Gerard while he was preparing to pick her up from the airport and told him that she was not coming back.

Gerard couldn't phone her back for an explanation, so he went to his Nana's to use her phone.

Nana, hovering in the background, witnessed the conversation and the devastation of her grandson. She clung to him, weeping. Her emotional response was difficult for Gerard to deal with, so he came around to me.

I answered the knock on the door and immediately saw Gerard's distress, his pale, shocked face.

'Mum,' he said, 'do you have room for me? Can I stay here?'

'You can have my breath if you need it,' I said.

Gerard slumped in a lounge chair and began to explain.

'Liane told me that she has left me. Just as I was putting on my shoes to get into the car to pick her up. Why did she wait to tell me? Was she planning this all along? I went to Nana to phone Liane, but Nana cried so much I couldn't think. I knew you would be calm and help me. I don't know what to do.'

Days turned into weeks. Gerard returned to their rented house and began a thorough clean-up. He regained emotional strength and confidence. He often picked me up in the mornings to go to Bunnings to get conduit and connections for his aquaponic project.

Gerard looked online for divorce proceedings. He downloaded divorce papers. He worked out and became fitter and healthier. I clung to the changes and hoped they would continue. He had reacted to Liane's job changes, dramatic fallout with friends, and partying and flirting. She had previously had an affair with

Gerard's best friend.

I didn't initiate any conversation about Liane. I knew Gerard would tell me what he felt was relevant. He told me he didn't know if there was someone else in the mix.

He had been approached by close friends who informed him that they believed Liane was having an affair with a mutual friend, a bloke known for promiscuity.

'I went around to visit those friends, and the bloke that was rumoured to be having a fling with Liane was there. He didn't like my attitude and pushed me. I pushed back and flattened him. I just can't believe Liane would have an affair with him. It was supposed to happen when she was babysitting our friends' children. How would that work?'

'People having affairs can be pretty creative,' I said, 'the thrill of the forbidden. Getting away with it.'

It was more than Gerard's mind could picture, so he was inclined to give Liane the benefit of the doubt.

Gerard had the long-distance capability restored on the phone. Liane refused to take his calls, then finally said she would return, but live with a friend.

Gerard's new confidence and independence evaporated.

'You're my everything,' he said to Liane.

The memory of these situations coloured my dread of them leaving. There was quiet mumbling about Perth. Western Australia was a long way, and I feared estrangement.

I was at their home less and less. When Flopsy Bunny and Mr Kitty were rehomed, I knew the inevitable.

Every time I came home from their place, Bronson would ask, 'Have you been voted off the island yet, Mum?'

'This time the island is leaving, Bronson.'

Bronson frowned. 'No more computer days with Gerard then. I love those.'

I had 11 months with my adorable granddaughter before Gerard and Liane packed up the house and left for West Australia, where Liane gave birth to two more children and where Gerard gained a job as a delivery driver and then driving trucks.

On one occasion, a heavy water tank fell on his head, and he was hospitalised for a concussion. Gerard thought he was fine and told the doctors that. He had thirteen clips on the top of his head and was told that only his thick neck and strong back had saved him.

For six gut-wrenching years, I had no contact.

I attended the memorial service for my brother in WA, nervous and hopeful that Gerard and his family were nearby, but I didn't see or hear from them. At the memorial, my sister-in-law had Peter's granddaughter read the piece I wrote and afterwards introduced me with, 'Linda is no good at funerals.'

Soon after, I heard that the family had moved to Brisbane. With no way to know how they were, I turned to a friend, also the mother of a close friend of Gerard and Liane, a mental health nurse whom I believed I could trust. She was my only hope of connection with my son. I phoned her, told her of my angst, the pain of separation, and my desperate desire to know how the family was going.

On her next visit, the woman related every word to Gerard and Liane. I was devastated.

Wilderness

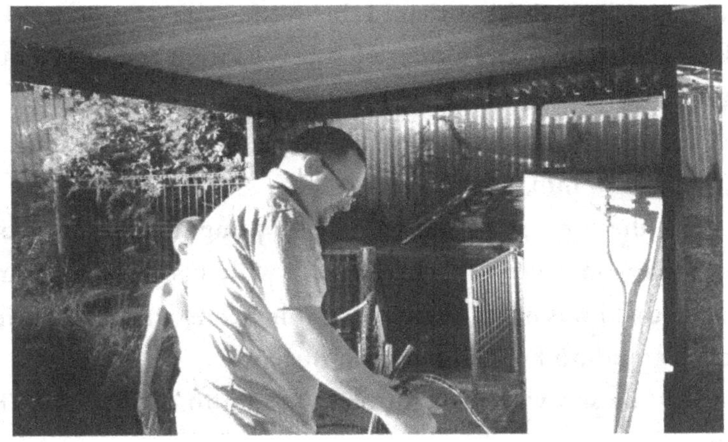

Throughout the estrangement, I was undone. I had failed. I couldn't communicate with my son. Couldn't reach him, know him.

Gerard was my firstborn, my 'only' for so long. The one I always said was Samuel, Hannah's son, as I read the story to him at bedtime. I told him that I would make him a coat every year that I drew breath, but I would never give him up to the Temple as Hannah did. I had made him a coat every year of his childhood and bought him a coat every year of his adult life.

He was the son who lived in and through my darkest days. And every day, a fresh apology on my lips that he shared my pain.

179

Always feeling that he never saw how much I knew his pain, as he fought and struggled against it, trying to protect three, not one.

He was the son whose name I screamed as he floundered in the cruel surf at Emerald Beach, so that someone else would hear, and do what I could not—swim out and save him from the rip that was taking him away. He was rescued that day by an off-duty lifesaver who was packing up to leave the beach. The man had been alerted by me screaming Gerard's name as I stood at the edge of the surf.

He was the son who aspired, dreamed, reached towards integrity, and sought to live without regrets. He came to embrace the concept of "tough love" that his beloved Uncle Gordon tried to instil, with his "I'll make a man of you yet", even though Gerard railed against it when he was young.

He was the son I would chase to heaven or hell for the sake of integrity if I saw him do wrong.

He was the son I struggled with, attempting to stop him from adding layer on layer of pain on me, with his inflexions and innuendo that I was not all I could be to him, constantly comparing me to his grandmother and her generous love.

He was the son who brought the question to my heart, "Who am I to you?"

I survived by reminding myself of the dimensions of my love: its surrender, its lonely-night heartache. I put my faith in the muscle memory of the heart. Gerard's heart.

And I waited. My son knew me. He would remember…

Returned to sender

You're here, with me

'I won't cry,' I said when I picked you up from the airport, broken. 'Thank you, Mum,' you said. 'If I cry, I won't stop.' You let me slip my hand through your strong arm. Whether it was for your comfort or mine, I don't know.

'It's not a long drive … home,' I said, flinching at the word home, for you were a long way from home. My home was no longer your home, but I didn't have another more suitable word.

I won't talk on the way … there,' I said, seeing gratitude in your eyes, those eyes identical to mine, eyes that began as blue, then slowly changed to hazel.

When you did feel like talking, your first subject was socks. 'Even took my socks,' you said, incredulous about the theft of socks.

Socks were a favourite subject thereafter. I watched as the lady at the bank, unfazed by your huge size, shaved head and bikie beard, stroked your hand.

'I'm autistic,' you told her, 'I miss a lot of cues. I didn't have socks. I miss my children.'

I flinched at your vulnerability, but this woman closed her hand over yours and said, 'It's going to be all right. You'll see.' You rewarded her with one of your warm smiles, warm eyes.

At the unemployment office, you quietly took over the computer when the counsellor couldn't work something out. He thanked you. It was ironic to be smarter than the guy helping.

I wondered at your willingness to have me with you everywhere you went. Was I safe? Was I home?

And just like when you were young, there were doctors: That annoying strabismus, surgery organised in Perth had not helped. Thyroid, GORD, hypertension, and, if those weren't enough, there was grieving and depression. The crippling feeling that had always followed you like a shadow, the spectre of failure, being misunderstood, unable to articulate "why".

You came with me everywhere and wanted me to be with you everywhere. Parallel play, just like when you were a kid.

When I developed an excruciating headache, you drove me to the doctor's and sat quietly. After we left, you said, 'Very generous of you, Mum. To offer the doctor three alternate diagnoses.'

'Oh, no. Did I really?'

You nodded.

I had trigeminal neuralgia, the first option I had given to the doctor.

I was surprised by your relief at the autism diagnosis, your only wish that it had been found earlier when your disconnect from people and the world first pained you. Typical of you, you read everything about autism that you could find, excited at the description of all those things that had held you back. The inability to cope with change at work, at home, and at school. You were angry that when I had taken you to psychologists, they had failed to see it, see your struggle, see you.

I fought Centrelink. Again. Fought for you to get on the disability pension after harassing civil servants and uncivil service providers. I wrote letters, focusing on Katherine Campbell (of Robodebt infamy).

You were sleeping soundly when someone phoned from Centrelink. They told you that your application had been approved.

You were astonished. 'Centrelink doesn't phone clients!' you said, 'you can't even phone them! I salute your letters, but I don't want to read them. There must have been a hundred of them in that pile.'

I shrugged.

'I'm as povvo as you now, Mum.'

We celebrated with chocolate.

Your physical strength, which had been a cornerstone of your identity, began to fail. Exhausted easily, you gave up swimming, a place of joy in former days. You tried the gym. We tried walking around the neighbourhood. The scrutiny and the weakening of your muscles scuttled that. You decreased medication, hoping for a return of strength.

You asked for your favourite meals, sighing with satisfaction at childhood favourites.

'We've only got food,' you said, devouring those "eggy things" I made. You would laugh at me today. I had a three-course breakfast. The kitchen is full of food, but empty of you.

In Brisbane, after seeing your three adoring children, a stomach bleed required hospitalisation. I raced you to Prince Charles Hospital at midnight, shoving aside my fear of traffic in a strange city. They sent you for a gastroscope. I sat eagerly at the waiting room door for your return, as I had done with your childhood surgeries.

When you returned to the ward, you were floating; that

marvellous anaesthetic drug had eased you into the tranquillity of a kind I had never seen you possess. It was like that Christmas when your stiff (possibly autistic) Grandmother drank alcoholic cider, resulting in a level of agreeableness never experienced before. Your uncle started to intervene, to warn her that the apple cider was alcoholic. You tapped him and said, 'Leave well enough alone, Uncle Pete.'

On the ward after the gastroscopy, you sat on the gurney, relaxed and talkative, surrounded by young nurses offering sandwiches and smiles. Several more girls came. Attracted to you, to your infectious smile and your 'yes, please'. I saw the way they looked at you. They saw a lovely big guy, an engaging guy and were drawn in. I don't think you believed me when I told you that. You'd never felt any kind of handsome.

I wanted to freeze time. I was if I was seeing you for the first time. Looking past your childhood awkwardness, that sombre boy with language far above his peers, those who called you "oddbod". You took that as a compliment, merely a statement of truth, and used it in your email address. That serious child with lost, hazel eyes.

The staff gave me your discharge summary. My heart sank to read "no reflexes, query cause".

Back in Adelaide, I took you to more doctors. To a doctor, who, with the name of Bing Wu, although looking Chinese, claimed to be Irish.

After the examination, he said that the symptoms suggested neurological, rather than muscular disease, proposing that the most likely diagnosis was Motor Neurone Disease. But the real test would be the rate of decline. He would know more on our next visit.

After another arduous GP session, you said, 'No more doctors,

Mum.'

I nodded.

I put a mattress along the hall so you could lean on it on the way to the bathroom when your legs failed you. Your body refused to obey. You stumbled, but never complained.

You got stuck on the toilet one night, alone, afraid. You called out to me, but I did not hear you. That haunts me still.

You can't call out to me again. You can't stumble and fall. The weakness of your body won't give you pain. You will never be alone or afraid again.

The hummingbird mother & you

We were never going to be a postcard family with reunion photos and carefully posed, perfectly poised memorabilia. Every photo I have is a moment caught in the everyday. Every photo has a story. The only time you posed beautifully was for a friend of mine.

I must have seemed chaotic to you. You with your flat affect, your plateau of sameness from day to day. You called me a hummingbird. While you struggled with the lows that had become your MO, I must have seemed frenetic at times.

'I don't understand you,' you said one time, with your belongings piled high in a trailer, leaving for the other side of the country. Further and further from me. You had come to say goodbye. Your adorable babe, then one year old, reached for me with both arms, leaning out of her mother's arms to come to Nana. 'You can't go to Nana,' your wife said, 'we're in a hurry.'

I reached for you then, desperate for connection and affirmation. 'Do you know yet when you'll forgive me?'

Forgive me for the man I married, the man who beat you to a pulp. Would you forgive me for staying after that, for living with the fear until there was a gap in the rage, a window, an opening?

While friends posted families with hundreds, we were there, in our small drama. Our disconnect.

There was always a time delay in telling me things. 'I didn't like…' and you'd tell me something that happened years before.

'You bring things to me,' I said, 'when it's too late for me to understand or fix. There's a five-year delay. (I had counted it out, you see). 'So I won't know for at least five years what you're thinking tonight. Could we change that? Could you shorten it? Tell me when it's now rather than brushed aside for a demi-decade?'

You grinned that quirky smile that usually preceded you calling me 'funny little mother'. The grin you had when your brother had done some daft thing, and you came around to the house, slapped him gently up the back of the head and said, 'Don't bring idiots into the house. She's my mother too, you know.'

It was dark when you drove off with the trailer packed high like something from the Beverly Hillbillies. You were chasing the next solution. Something that would change the struggle of your days. A new start. I had lost count of them. Watched them as they failed. Because the out-of-sync disconnect was within you. The dull lingering thuds of autism. You gave it other names. Attached it to people. This is to blame. That is to blame.

You were never going to fit in some of those places. You worked the night shift at the factory. Your boss was "a dick". You offered him the respect that he deserved. None. One night he had sidled up to you and said, 'Your mother is a bit of alright.'

Others might have shrugged it off. Not you. You leaned towards him with your big bulk and said, 'If you ever mention my mother again, I'll throw you down.' His wife left him later, shattered and afraid, domestic violence.

I saw the small swells of enthusiasm as you undertook each new thing, new job, new study. Then saw the change. Change, that enemy of yours. You were going so well as manager of a pizza place.

Your calm self-possession, attention to detail and your devotion to The Rules, the Formula, excellent qualities for the job. It was going so well, until it wasn't. Until the owner wanted you to go to a new location. Oversee the setting-up for the new pizza place. You just left. Never explaining. Because you didn't know that the shadow of dislocation was part of your autism. We later talked about how different things would have been if you could have articulated the acute discomfort of The New.

After the Wilderness Years, the years of my exile from you, when you came back to live with me, our world was a different place. After a few days of settling in, back living with your mother, the hummingbird, you said to me, 'I don't like that, Mum. Please don't do it again.'

'Praise the Lord,' I said, 'you've shortened the five-year gap. Thank you. I can't navigate our relationship if you withhold the map.'

'Don't get too carried away, Mum.'

How I had longed for your words, so carefully constructed. How many times have I sat with you in some café, waiting for you to open up and tell me about your world? Thinking I would understand better, never knowing that you had no idea yourself. You were waiting for words and understanding just as I was.

I remember the year when you had no money for my birthday, and I said, 'Words will do. The gift of words will do. Tell me something I did right as a mother. That will be better than any other present.'

'You were really good when I vomited,' you said.

'I'll take it,' I said.

'Can I have the car, please, Mum. I'm going to file for divorce. I have to go to the court to file the papers.'

'Do you want me to come?'

'No mother. My brother is coming with me. He's applying for a marriage license, and before you say it, yes, I do see the irony.'

Off they went, my two sons, on an ordinary Wednesday, grinning similar grins. The big calm guy with his chatty brother.

When you came home, you told me one of your stories.

'You won't believe what the mad boy did, Mum!'

I smiled. I was usually the protagonist in the stories between brothers.

'We walked in the doors of the court and the boy turned around and legged it. I was left standing there like a goose. Didn't know what was going on. Turns out he was carrying a pocket knife, and when he saw the security guards he realised.'

'That'd be right. He's into all that survival stuff. Carries the damn thing everywhere. I'm always worried he'll get arrested.'

'Don't be silly, Mum. Not with that baby face he won't.'

We looked into what we called "Government Stuff & Nonsense". The paperwork that was necessary to uphold your autism diagnosis and gain the right kind of help. You had been diagnosed by a psychologist in Brisbane, called "someone or other". As hard as you tried, you couldn't remember the name, but remembered the clinic. So we chased that up, and down. You had seen a specialist psychiatrist in the city. You couldn't remember his name either.

'It's a weird name, Mum. Very long surname. Thirteen syllables.'

That specialist became "Dr Thirteen Syllables". Dr Thirteen Syllables said this. Dr Thirteen Syllables said that.

I turned to Tony Attwood, the friend who had contributed to the first two books. We visited him, went through the process for the third time, and after I took up the cudgels with Centrelink et al., we finally gained recognition.

You were thrilled to meet Tony Attwood. During the two-hour consult, Tony talked about "Callan the Chameleon," the children's book that we co-authored.

I rattled on about something.

'It's not about you, Mum,' you said.

You made a new best friend in the small country town where I had bought a house near your brother. Cindy, the lady at the takeaway. You would sit on the barstool while she prepared your burger and chips, and you talked. You had found your words. Your understanding of yourself. 'I'm autistic,' you said, and she nodded, grateful for your willingness to open up.

'I was angry when they told me. Apparently, that's part of it. Went with the wife to get my son tested. They mentioned all the things they thought were odd, different about him, and I said, "What's wrong with that – I do all those things". And then they looked at me. Wow. I went home and read everything I could find. I read the list of symptoms they had given me to help with my son. It was a description of me, of how I felt, how I acted and reacted. I was so angry. When I got to the last thing on the list, it explained that anger was the usual response. Then I knew. I'm autistic. How different my life could have been. The work discomfort. The inability to accept change. Shutting down in big groups.'

Every day you had new words. New understandings. You hadn't been holding your words against your chest, refusing to share them, unwilling to let someone in. You didn't have the words. Until you did.

Over lettuce and beetroot, fried egg and cheese, you nattered. You shared with Cindy about your heartache over losing your wife and children. And she shared about her divorce, the crippling anxiety and the joy of finding love again with a wonderful man, encouraging you to hope, to live again.

Hope grew. But hope was dependent on your children. And that made hope a precarious thing indeed.

I sometimes went with you. I became fond of the takeaway girls too. I sometimes went alone.

One day, Cindy said to me, 'That boy thinks the world of you!'

I felt my heart swell. All the dearth of the past years was swept away. You didn't just love me, you thought the world of me, your funny little hummingbird mother.

I went home and told you what Cindy had said.

'You could have told me that,' I said, hopeful of words from the horse's mouth, but you grinned, that most excellent grin.

'Well, now you know,' you said, as if I had all that I needed.

Here instead of there

Some of these stories are things Gerard said, stories he told, usually over tea with his brother and his brother's wife, where the conversation would begin with: 'Let me tell you the mad thing Mum did this week.'

Here, in the book, sometimes I have written TO him.

And at other times, I have written stories in his voice. Just as he told them to me. We thought alike. We wrote alike.

Then there are the other stories, the ones where he was attempting to fit the jigsaw pieces of the puzzle of his life together through the complex lens of his autism.

For these, I have written in his voice, as the one who knew him best at the time, as his mother, his carer, his confidante, and friend.

In Gerard's voice...

Off The Plane

there's mum
standing so still
as her eyes
zigzag
back and forth
looking for me.

she sees me,
moves toward the end
of the ramp. She doesn't swamp, crush
me with hugs, she just puts
her arm through mine and says,
'It's okay. I'm not going to cry.'
'I'm glad,' I say, 'because I'll cry too.'

she leads me to car, quietly. I throw the suitcase
in the boot. She says, 'I'll take you home.'
But she can't take me home. I don't have a home.
Mum sighs, 'sorry,' she says.

home walked out the door, leaving
me with a mattress, a bowl, a plate
and misery. I took more tablets then
begging the pain to stop. My wife,
My children. My life. Everything.
Gone.

Going ... there

In the car Mum tries to show me some of the new clothes she bought for me.

I close my eyes. I don't care. 'Thanks,' I say, 'later.'

Mum tells me about the help she's lined up. I need it and want it, but I can't listen now. She pats my arm and drives in silence.

Mum gives me fat chunky pillows, pillows I keep and use every night. They're just right, in this nothing is right world in which I now live. Mum's flat could be anywhere, anything.

I don't know if its here or there. I only know it is empty of my wife, my children.

I sleep. Sleep is the only time the nightmare stops. I pray that I won't dream. I shiver in shock, wake up in a sweat, then shower. Back to sleep, there's a warm pressure on my chest.

Mum is checking up on me, hoping she doesn't wake me, remembering what a heavy sleeper I used to be but am no longer. Sleep is an indifferent presence, an unpredictable commodity.

Mum's Sad Eyes are hard to watch, when she looks in the suitcase for clothes. I tell her I have none, but I guess she didn't know how bad things were. How little I have.

Mum wants to throw them all out, and I don't care until she picks up a pair of socks, 'Not them,' I say, 'John gave me those.'

'Good old John,' she says, 'and Joy.

I'm awake now, and I want to talk. Talk about everything because if I can just line things up, then I might start to make sense of it all. I tell her I only have the Op Shop clothes I found in a bin at the hospital when I talked the staff into letting me go. I had no money for the train fare. My wife wouldn't pick me up. I shouldn't have been surprised; she only brought my oldest daughter in once to see me, while she sat texting, bouncing her foot, the way she does when she's agitated.

When I arrived at the hospital, they asked if I took drugs and didn't believe me until the blood test results came back. They asked about violence – I'm a big guy and look rough. That's been useful a time or two. Sometimes not.

On the train ride from the Caboolture Hospital, back to the house, my size did me no favours.

A bloke sitting near me freaked out, moved away, and sat further down the carriage. He left his wallet on the seat. I tapped him on the shoulder. He jerked when he saw me. 'Sorry mate,' I said, 'you left this on the seat.'

He was relieved then, said 'Thanks,' and something like, 'Not many people would do that, mate.'

I was worried about ticket checkers. I didn't have a ticket, but no one came, which was just as well because I didn't have a clue what to say.

I've never been anywhere as empty as that house was without my family.

I didn't even look for my stuff.

I looked for the kids' things. I found a few of their toys and put them in a box, found a marker pen and wrote 'Treasures' on the box. It was as if the place had been cleaned out in a hurry, because no one would have wanted my undies and socks. Leaving me not one pair of socks.

Why my clothes? Why socks? Why me?

My tools had been disappearing for a while. My wife had even helped me look for them, but now I realise that was a pretence. All those eBay accounts, furtive transactions, blasé explanations.

Optimism

There are times when I'm almost optimistic, and I've never been good at optimism. I line things up in my head. How things will be when my wife lets me come home, when she's done holding me at a distance, waiting for me to learn whatever it is I'm supposed to learn, and changing whatever it is she wants changed.

I can never work out what she wants from me.

It seems to be obvious to everyone but me. She wanted me to stay at home, look after the kids, so she could go to work, study and all that.

I know how Mum feels. She's expecting me to fall out of love soon, not knowing that I can't. She's holding back, as best as Mum can hold back. When I tell her stuff about Liane, she says, 'Hmm,' then 'Sure about that?'

'Whatdya mean?' I say.

'Is it the truth?'

'I dunno how to tell.'

'If she's breathing, that's how.'

My wife will never forgive me for going to Mum. I care less about that as the days go by.

Mum's Got A Bee In Her Bonnet

Mum doesn't know that I know what she's up to. Doesn't know that I watch her, cup of tea in one hand, pruning shears in the other, humming to herself as she clips the hedge that's been bothering her. 'Have you got permission to do that?' I ask. 'You're a tenant.'

'Course I have,' she says, sipping her tea.

After she's clipped enough to clear the path to make it safe and clean out the rats' nests, she realises that she's fixed one problem and created another. What is left behind looks like an ancient trap from King Arthur's time. It's all spikes.

'Fuck it,' she says, 'I'll have to take more.'

I tell Bronson that she should give up.

He grins. 'She should've given up before she started, but you know Mum.' He tries to have the same conversation with her, but she pulls out her phone and shows him the messages to and from the CEO of the corporate body. Then she blahs on about Jason, the yard maintenance guy and how bothered he is by the hedge, how his wife is doing with the cancer, how the CEO bloke bought a bookshelf when she invited him in. 'How the blazes do you know all that stuff?' he asks her.

'People talk to me,' she says, like she's normal or something, which is highly debatable.

Bronson turns to me and says, 'she gets out of as much trouble as she gets into, you know,' as if I didn't know after being around her for a heck of a lot longer than him.

So then it's a daily joke with Bronson. We talk over the fence. He checks out Mum's progress, grins, and, like me, waits for the shit to hit the fan. It doesn't take long. The old duck opposite, the one who screams at everyone who walks on the lawn, takes the first shot. She hunts Mum down and gets stuck in. Daft cow.

'You were complaining about it last week,' says Mum—this only gets the old girl worked up, and she threatens to phone the CEO. 'Off you go then,' says Mum.

That's when the fun really starts.

The old girl's daughter gets stuck into Mum and gets a sharp, comprehensive lecture from Mum on the government regulations about rat infestations and health that Mum googled.

The silly bitch says, 'They're native fruit rats.'

That really sends Bronson and me right over the edge. We're starting to enjoy this nonsense. Neither of us worries about Mum, but we're a bit concerned we'll get the blame because who is going to believe that Mum has managed to prune a ten metre stretch of hedge that the yard maintenance guy baulked at?

There are tonnes of green waste on the lawn.

I think it's about time to talk to Mum about gravity. She's looking a bit sheepish by now because she's had to cut the hedge right back to the brick fence because of the sharp twigs. It's a magnificent mess.

The weight of the hedge that's left starts to lean. Then lean some more. It's a matter of time. I'm watching this bit with great anticipation because the guy who owns the house where all that heavy hedge is headed holds loud parties that start just after lunchtime on a Sunday and go on all bloody night. They're outdoor parties with drunk yobbos singing along to loud doof doof music. I've often said I'd like to throw something over the fence, but it looks like gravity, and Mum will provide just that.

The inevitable happens. Without the weight from this side of the fence to balance it, the hedge falls. The party idiot next door no longer has a backyard, a side yard, or privacy. He joins the lengthening queue at the door to take a potshot at Mum.

I'd feel sorry for him if he wasn't such a dick.

'Hello,' says Mum, smiling, 'you're here to yell at me too.'

I sit around the corner. This is too good to miss. The guy rambles about damage and devastation, then moves on to his treasured, but now forever lost, privacy. And that's his second mistake. Tackling Mum being the first. 'Privacy!' she says, 'privacy! You care about your privacy when you regularly destroy the privacy of the whole street with your all-night parties. I must be odd because I would have thought that people who value privacy would not have drunken outdoor karaoke for all the world to hear.'

The guy's shoulders sag. I don't think he's thought of his parties as drunken outdoor karaoke. He mutters about having a few noise complaints, anonymous notes in the letterbox, that sort of thing.

'I don't do anonymous,' says Mum.

There are no more parties.

There's a minuscule area of his yard in the middle of the green carnage where Mr Privacy sits at a small table under an umbrella in the rain, reading the newspaper and sipping his coffee alone. It's a sight of such rare pleasure and satisfaction that I walk past often, stare over the fence for the sole purpose of enjoying the sight.

Those three years

Are you still here?

From the time Gerard returned until his death, I watched over him as he slept. At first, he slept in the loungeroom where I had a single bed that served as a couch.

I would walk softly to him as he lay on his back. I would place my hand on his chest, ever so gently, to see if he was breathing.

He had been a heavy sleeper before, teased by his friends who had tried to wake him on occasion, even dragging him onto the slate floor while he slept on.

But every time I placed my hand on his chest, he woke. 'What, Mum?'

I never explained, just said a quick 'sorry' and made a hasty retreat. I kept doing it. I couldn't see his chest move, couldn't hear his soft breathing. He endured this without reproach.

We didn't have to wait long for mental health. One of my friends was a psychiatrist, and he sorted hospital-based psychiatric visits, where Gerard's medications were monitored and prescribed.

A psychologist, a mental health worker and then the whole job-seeking malarkey, where Gerard had to step in and show the counsellor how to use the computer program and the printer.

'You can have my job,' said the counsellor, smiling.

'No thanks,' said Gerard, 'too much whingeing for me.'

'You don't whinge,' said the counsellor.

'Yeah, but I'm weird.'

As winter arrived to replace the heat of summer, Gerard needed new clothes. He'd arrived with nothing but what he was wearing, old things he had garnered from the hospital bin.

Gerard begrudgingly came shopping for clothes a few times but chose to give me money to buy them. I purchased sleep shorts and T-shirts. Board shorts and cargo shorts. A pair of jeans, hoodies.

The cargo shorts never saw the light of day because Gerard wore the sleep shorts everywhere. He hardly ever wore long pants, and one pair of jeans took care of that.

He had always been drawn to clothes that didn't draw attention, but he saw me looking at a website for colourful hippy-style jackets. 'I'll have one of those. That one,' he said, walking to his room to transfer money to my account to pay for it.

An Akubra came next, on special order for the largest size they made. Any remarks I made on how this explained my need for a caesarean birth were greeted with, 'Mother! Really? Nobody wants to hear that.'

Mr Clooney

'A fire needs a cat,' said Gerard as we sat and watched the flames in the wood heater, in the new house, as we relished the heat. He brought the cat subject up several times over the next few days. I looked on Gumtree and fell in love with every kitten and cat I saw.

'I want a ginger cat,' I said.

We made concrete plans. Bronson told us that the Animal Welfare place was the place to go. I bought a carrier, and we headed off to the rescue centre, with Gerard driving.

The lady at the desk gave us the drill. 'We like you to spend at least half an hour with a prospective pet.'

Gerard stood back while I approached the cages.

A ginger kitten climbed a stick that was leaning against the grid wire. It rubbed against my hand and purred.

'This one,' I said, opening the door to pick him up.

'Mum. We can't go yet. The lady said to take half an hour.'

'Oh tosh,' I said, 'this one chose me. Who am I to question fate?'

'You'll have to think of a name then.'

'Mr Clooney,' I said, remembering all the times I had warned Bronson not to somersault into my bed because one day he would land on George Clooney.

On the way home in the car, Mr Clooney threw up, wet himself and pooed. He trembled and meowed tiny mewling sounds.

Gerard wound the window down. 'Well, at least we know that all his orifices work.'

When we arrived back home, Gerard shrugged on a coat.

'I'm off to the Gungellan,' he said, then decided to give me some feline advice even though I had owned more cats than he ever had. 'Now, Mum. It will take days for the kitten to get used to the place and to get close to you, so don't be disappointed if he hides for a bit. A few days even.'

When Gerard came home from the pub with his appetite sated, he was surprised to see tiny Mr Clooney asleep on my shoulder.

Gerard had had several cats before, and I thought he would enjoy patting our new kitten, but his OCD had gone up a notch, and he was compulsively washing his hands. He couldn't pet Mr Clooney with his hands, but he stroked the kitten with his foot, which the kitten enjoyed and emitted a soft moan. So we called this mode of affection "oof pats".

Mr Clooney squeaked rather than meowed. I claimed he had half a voice box. Bronson and his wife's cat had a meow that pierced ears and broke eardrums. I was perfectly content with my quiet, zen little puss, especially as he showed no sign of wanting to climb and destroy curtains or furniture, happy to scratch at a cat post, where he often stretched out.

I had many misadventures with Mr Clooney. If I couldn't find him, I wandered the yard weeping like a paid mourner.

This nonsense was told and retold over dinner whenever Bronson and Bella came over.

Mr Clooney sleeps at the bottom of my bed after head-butting me gently in order to receive pats and scratches. He is a balm, a companion, untouched by the loneliness that sometimes haunts my days. I watch over him like a mother hen, afraid of losing him.

The corn-row doctor

The waiting room is too small. The lights too bright, a thousand watts or more, lasering tired eyes and flimsy nerves. The outdoors too near, more inside than out. You can see half the town, people walking, dogs with heads on paws resigned to long waits on leashes, eyebrows flinching. The place is a goldfish bowl, for guppies seeking to linger, kissing glass edges, eyeing humans and pondering what made them stare at fish in bowls.

The chairs are too close together, rooms too close to each other. The people are strange with no sense of order, or queuing. No respect for silence or smells or loud scrapings. Sniffing and coughing, gouging out what's left of the quiet. Clanking, squeaking toys lie on noise enhancing floor. There's an infant with superhuman strength, banging and thumping toys that rattle with metallic exuberance, clatter and deafen, shredding nerves. The floor is too noisy with its linoleum cheapness, its fierce economy and insulting thinness, a poor skin for cement, hard, cold. There are too many doors hiding hallways and corridors, with heels smacking down, while echoes chase echoes. The receptionist's desk is too high and remote with the tired, sick and miserable far below, seeking comfort and quiet yet forced to yell symptoms and diseases to brisk secretaries who then find patient records that guarantee "privacy". But what's the use of that when she asks, 'Why are you here? Why do you want the doctor?

Did she expect some to say, 'it's just a social call, I was just passing and thought I'd drop by'?

But no, poor old gents lean forward with hoarse whispers and mutters. 'I'm having troubling whizzing'. But she can't hear and asks again. So phlegm-scratching cough and the old man repeats a bit louder, 'I can't take a piss', then subsides into silence and shrugs at his wife, who's scanning the room for magazines and wondering if she's read that New Idea, or not.

There are stupid conversations on the right and the left.

A sneezing old man with rampant nose hair sits too close, wet, germ-soaked handkerchief tucked in a pocket, not retreating. The kid with the toy with coloured balls on curved wires bashes it again and again on the floor, then, when his mother stops this satisfying activity, he screams louder than toys until she gives it back and it begins again, the screech and thundering. There's a sign on the wall that offers false promise—"Wait Time: no longer than 20 minutes". The chairs are lined up the wrong way, like seats on a bus. A doctor comes out of the room opposite. No, please not him, he looks like an unkempt gardener who couldn't tend a row of beans. How will he know about the subtleties of mental trauma? He doesn't seem careful, so how could he care about people and maladies that belong in the head but fall out, run around, create havoc and can't be tamed, corralled or ridden – get back in the saddle.

The unkempt man calls out.

My son, Gerard rises. Oh bother, it's for him, for us.

Inside the unkempt doctor asks questions so puerile and inane that I wonder if this is all a practical joke and perhaps he is the gardener. The platitudes come quickly. 'Were you bullied at school? he asks, not solemnly but with curiosity more common in bored housewives or persons undertaking indifferent surveys on street corners.

'Yes', says my son. 'Weren't we all?'

'What happened for that to stop?' asks the unkempt doctor.

'I grew,' says Gerard.

Unkempt doctor asks 'What's worrying you today?'

'Coming here, doing this, police,' says Gerard.

'Ah!' the unkempt doctor pounces, staring down his narrow nose, 'why the police?' he asks, eagerly eyeing the mountain as if the gentle man in front of him might have been tempted to gang bash someone or do a ram raid if he had time, but my son meekly says, 'You get fined $500 for not wearing a seatbelt in this state.'

The doctor sighs. He's disappointed. He has a dull job. This intrusive dill continues pushing his questions as if my son is docile, dim and poorly presented, not knowing the huge patience and kind-heartedness, definitely not the intelligence.

I know my son is struggling to work out if the problem is with him, or the doctor.

When we leave Gerard drives, he's very quiet, cogitating.

I can't take any more.

'That bloody doctor. He's an idiot. We're never going there again, not for that condescension, that patronising git of man.'

Gerard heaves a sigh. 'That's a relief. I thought it was me.' He mutters, 'I couldn't decide if he was going to go bald or not.'

I laugh. I explain that the unkempt doctor has had plastic surgery, hair transplants. I explain the procedure, the slits, the transfer, the mapped precision.

Gerard is amazed and touches his shaved head. 'That explains the rows, the symmetry,' he says. 'There he is telling me not to be anxious about life and he can't cope with losing a bit of hair.'

'I know,' I say, 'the irony.'

It's only been half an hour but it seems like six months. I've walked in his shoes, maybe one mile or two. I've been hyper-stimulated, noise confronted, confused, insulted, misunderstood and bemused – an autistic nightmare.

I don't much like it. I don't know how Gerard does this. Day after day.

Gerard meets Tony Attwood

Gerard had been diagnosed in Brisbane by a psychiatrist, whose name he couldn't remember, whom we referred to as Doctor 13 syllables.

Gerard told me the name of his general practitioner, and we started from there for him to get the diagnosis made official to the standard required by Centrelink. The records we obtained from his GP were not deemed sufficient.

In South Australia at the time, the usual route for diagnosis was through a psychologist or speech therapist, and it was only available to children. Adults were supposed to attend a psychiatrist, but only one of three was on the official list. Gerard had attended two psychiatrists who specialised in autism since his arrival in SA, but neither of their assessments was acceptable. When I checked with the three designated psychiatrists, they were unavailable.

Gerard had been seeing a psychologist in Glenelg for over a year, and this was also insufficient. This was incredibly frustrating. Gerard was keen to have an official, acceptable diagnosis.

I had met Tony Attwood when I was writing *I'm not broken, I'm just different*. We had exchanged books, and he had loved the children's book, *Callan the Chameleon*. Gerard was thrilled at the prospect of meeting Tony. Foremost in his thoughts was the possibility that he might also be able to get some assistance from

Tony for his small son, whose diagnosis had thrust Gerard into a realisation of his own autism.

Gerard was excited about getting an appointment with Tony. 'I will be happy to tell him anything.'

'Gerard, you tell everyone you meet you're autistic!' I said.

'Yeah.' He grinned. 'I don't care about that. I want everyone to know so that they don't have false expectations about me and that they begin to understand me and understand autism.'

I phoned Tony's secretary, made an appointment and prepared for the trip to Brisbane, coinciding with his court appearance for custody and access. Gerard went back and forth with his wife, trying to arrange visitation. She was sceptical, so I spoke with her and sent her the confirmation email of Gerard's appointment with Tony.

Gerard was struggling with all the paperwork, so he asked me to help him fill out the lengthy forms to send to Tony prior to the interview.

'What do you mean *help*, Gerard?'

He sighed theatrically, leaned back in the chair, a habit that always freaked me out, but he never tipped over. He smiled a smug smile and said, 'You're better at this stuff than me and besides, you can't stop yourself.'

'I don't want to taint or influence your answers.'

'Don't be daft, Mum. How could you ever do that? You're always saying I don't take any notice of what you say.'

I read the questions while he relaxed back, his hands locked behind his head as he looked at the ceiling, carefully considering his answers and answering far more swiftly than I would have done on a similar assessment.

'Thanks, Mum.'

The rest was a nightmare. Gerard resisted the clothes I wanted him to wear. All preparations for the trip were arduous.

'You look like a homeless person,' I said, 'or a gangster.'

'Yeah,' he said, smiling, 'kinda what I was going for.'

'But you'll be in family court. That's not a good look for a father. Your wife's new bloke will be spiffed up. She'll make sure of that, and by comparison...'

'I don't do "comparison". It's who I am, and I wish you'd let it go. I'm not going to a barber to have my beard trimmed. I'm not wearing uncomfortable, hot clothes or fancy shoes. This is all hard enough, Mum.'

'I think the judge does "comparison",' I said, but Gerard had already left the room for a much-needed break from his overbearing mother.

The whole cloud of going to family court, seeing his ex-wife, her new husband and the children, overshadowed any anxiety about the flight and the mundane arrangements. Gerard was slow to respond to everything apart from transferring his share of the flight cost to my account.

On the day of our departure, Gerard seemed unaware of the concept of "time" and meandered and procrastinated until I was as overwhelmed as he was. I was the one driving to the airport, even though Gerard usually drove and was better at it than I was. I would leave the car there.

I had given Gerard a very specific time that allowed for all contingencies. I reminded him every five minutes.

He was late. I panicked.

As I opened the door, Mr Clooney, also agitated by all the fuss, chose that time to escape the chaos and loped out the door.

I fought the urge to lie in the foetal position and cry.

We could not look for the cat. We could not wait for Mr Clooney to decide to return to hearth and home. We didn't have time. I was miserable at the thought of losing my kitty.

So we left.

'Ring your brother,' I said crossly when we were in the car.

'What for?'

'Tell him about Mr Clooney. He'll have to…'

'Jeez, Mum. I'll do it later.'

I jumped up and down in the seat. I know this sounds weird to achieve while driving, but trust me, it's possible.

'For crying out loud, Gerard. For once in your miserable life, do something the first time you're asked.' Angry tears fell, and expletives were uttered. By me.

Gerard pulled his phone out. 'Hey,' he said to Bronson. 'Cat got out. You know what to do.'

I heard a 'yeah, good luck, Deddor' from the other end. "Deddor" being the name Bronson called his older brother before he could handle a G sound.

Gerard put the seat back and shut his eyes while I stressed about one of my least favourite things in life, driving through city traffic.

At the airport, Gerard was efficiency itself. Asking for help. Carrying all the bags. He flicked them effortlessly onto the conveyor as if he did it every day. He scanned stuff and did things with the Q cards I had bought, but didn't understand.

Then we did one of his favourite things and ate. I was sure I couldn't eat a thing due to my stomach being in knots, but I found that I enjoyed it as much as he did.

'We only have food, Mum,' he said, a new phrase he repeated to cover the fact that everything else in his life had disappeared.

At Tony's, we were welcomed warmly. Half the cost of the appointment was put through my medical fund, as I wanted to converse with Tony too.

With his big, beautiful smile, Gerard shook Tony's hand and charmed the man instantly. He then slouched in the chair to demonstrate his comfort with the situation and his trust, perhaps in me, surely in Tony.

Gerard was wearing pyjama shorts that he swore blind looked just like any other shorts. I worried that he might turn up to court like that, but put it aside as Tony began.

I told Tony that I didn't understand how Gerard had gained a high distinction in Philosophy at Uni. I assumed that it was the last subject that would suit an autistic person.

'Critical thinking and reason are his native language,' Tony said.

Gerard smiled, clearly enjoying having someone understand him implicitly and meaning he didn't have to say anything. But whenever I said anything else, Gerard turned to me and said, 'It isn't about you, Mum.'

If I hadn't been on my best behaviour, I would have outlined all the ways that proved that it was also about me.

Gerard, relieved that he was being seen and heard, had no trouble opening up to Tony.

After explaining the results of the assessment forms and their early conversation, Tony said, 'Congratulations, you have autism, Level One.'

Tony then posed a question to Gerard. 'Who are you?'

I expected Gerard to have a list ready, but he simply said, 'I don't know.'

I was shocked. I opened my mouth to fill the gap and give some prompts, but shut it again. This bit wasn't about me.

Tony brought out a huge sheet of paper and a Sharpie and made the list that Gerard could not. Strengths. Qualities.

Seeing my son so at ease brought tears to my eyes.

Tony gave Gerard a DVD of the 2-hour interview and the chart he had done with Gerard on regaining self-esteem.

Back at Joy and John's, where we were staying, Joy grinned and showed Gerard the large packet of Coco Pops she had bought.

'Ace,' said Gerard.

Gerard's wife arrived with his three children.

She filled the room, instantly comfortable and chatty. She introduced the new husband, who smiled shyly and avoided the mountain that was Gerard.

Gerard had no intention of cooperating with introductions, gave the bloke the side-eye and was soon wrapped in the arms of his girls, while his son clung to his mother and peeked at the new environment and people with apprehension.

Joy, ever the earth mother, chatted with Gerard's wife and soon had the youngest two diverted and playing with toys, while the oldest, Daddy's girl, clung to Gerard, afraid to ever let him go again.

Q&A for Tony Attwood

I've written much about autism, but I'm only ever fumbling around from the outside, often waiting for explanations that don't come easily. In order to connect with Gerard, I would take him out to lunch at a café where we could have milkshakes and hot chips. I would sit back and hope for a casual conversation to reveal his inner thoughts. 'Great chips, Mum. Thanks.'

I watched all manner of movies that I would not have chosen in a million years. Conan the Barbarian and other mind-numbing offerings. Gerard didn't open up. I did. I gave a sarcastic commentary. Gerard never told me that I was spoiling the movie. Never told me to shut up. I still don't know what he thought of my ramblings.

When I made the appointment for him with Tony Attwood, Gerard wrote a list of things that made up his life experiences. He couldn't be bothered using a capital for i. It was revealing to say the least. So if you want a taste of how the autistic mind works….

"In year 3 at school we were playing pin the tail on the donkey and a friend of mine was the furthest from the mark, kids were laughing at him so he said it was my tail so they laughed at me.

I never forgave him for that.

I go over conversations i haven't yet had or that i have already had over and over in my head.

At no point that i can remember was i susceptible to peer pressure. If i felt pressured, even in late teens, i would leave. I was proud of the fact my friends would tell others that came into the group from time to time 'don't try and force him'.

I remember being taken to places and being upset that i was out, even if i knew the people.

If i was sent to my room as punishment i saw this a good thing.

I was always anxious, especially if it might be likely that i would be the centre of attention and be embarrassed. it was sometimes so bad i would vomit.

I would rather play by myself at home than with friends.

I had good mimicking skills. Other kids or teachers.

I hated parties, organised games.

I was good at sport but i didn't want to do it because you got congratulated.

I didn't like getting gifts because you were then supposed to like and be grateful for the gift, even if it was a pair of scratchy woollen socks. I only like 100% cotton clothes, otherwise the sensation of wearing them is unbearable.

I have always liked to chew ice, i like the temperature sensation.

I really really hated it when my friends would introduce me to ppl they knew and expect that they would then be allowed into our group of friends.

I can't sleep unless the room is dark with no lights and no sound.

I can't concentrate if there is a lot going on, movement and sounds, ie., if my kids were all yelling and my ex was cranky about something i couldn't deal with any of it, i would have to remove myself from the room.

I can't tell if someone is angry or sad without verbal explanation.

When i was young and even later in life i like someone else to be in the house but not necessarily in the same room."

Family Court

In the Family Court carpark, Gerard jettisoned the casual blazer I bought him.

I frowned and sighed. He was wearing shorts, proper shorts. He wore his old, comfortable sneakers. He'd trimmed his beard. He answered my sideways glance with, 'It's hot. It's Brisbane.'

We met Gerard's solicitor and barrister. The solicitor could have easily sold real estate for the way he made promises and explained heck knows what. I didn't believe him, but Gerard hung on his every word and committed everything to memory.

The barrister was a more sophisticated and measured kind of guy. 'Can't make promises,' he said, 'it's an uphill battle. You're unemployed and struggling with depression. You've got limited financial resources, and you don't have ideal living conditions of a separate room for all the kids if they come to South Australia.'

Inside the courtroom, the barrister seemed overwhelmed. Perhaps he realised what a steep hill Gerard had to climb to gain custody. Gerard didn't have employment, lived with his mother in a two-bedroom home and had been hospitalised for a suicide attempt.

The same couldn't be said for the solicitor for Liane. She performed like a television star.

I realised what Gerard was up against, and all the confident ramblings of Gerard's solicitor were hollow words.

Family counselling was arranged. This gave Gerard hope.

We flew back to Brisbane for the family counselling. All three children participated, and I was required to attend.

The children behaved beautifully. Liane's husband and new baby were there in a separate room with an adjoining door. The new baby was quiet and happy.

The children went from being with Gerard and me to being with Liane. While Gerard was in with the counsellor, Marlow fretted for his mother, so I opened the adjoining door and said, 'Hello, that baby is so good. She hasn't cried once.'

Liane and I chatted about the baby and Marlow, Daisy and Lee.

The children now had one large room and wandered back and forth.

Gerard came out and wasn't entirely comfortable with the new arrangement.

It was my turn to go in.

The counsellor, as well as asking questions about Gerard and the children, expressed concern about what I was taking on if Gerard gained custody.

When she talked about Gerard, I got a sinking feeling that she would not support his quest for custody, despite the children's angst, especially Daisy's.

Unfortunately, Gerard had been unable to clearly articulate his thoughts and desires, but had relied on pages and pages of reports and notes, rather than expressing things in words. Even with encouragement, he had been unable to give up his sheets of paper, thinking that they were the key to his success.

I don't have enough percents.

The weekend after court, Gerard's three children came to stay with us. Eight, six and four. Daisy, the oldest clung to Gerard like a limpet in a rockpool, begging for airfare prices, planes to catch, luggage to pack, ways to be with her father.

Marlow, the middle child, Gerard's autistic son, had trouble relating to anyone other than Gerard and his older sister. He suffered from a speech delay, and Daisy encouraged him in his speech and protected him like a mother hen.

While Daisy wouldn't let Gerard out of her sight and Lee was interrogating me, Gerard's son lay surrounded by tech toys that he had rejected in preference for my iPad, which he quietly informed me didn't have enough per cent. Pointing to the top-right corner of the device to demonstrate, tilting his head without making eye contact, hoping this new, strange person understood percents. After all, this new person had loaned the iPad, that marvellous thing he had desired for his entire short life. It didn't take him long to run out of "percents".

I fetched the charger and plugged it in. He gazed at the top of my head, 'Shanks you,' he said, teasing a salty tear to my eyes at the careful politeness. So like Gerard. Yet not like Gerard, without Gerard's professorial speech and advanced vocabulary. Marlow curled into the mattress on the floor, alone, absorbed in his own world while his sisters connected to anyone and everyone.

Daisy, while keeping a vigilant eye on her beloved father, still managed to corral and chasten the younger two, tolerating their slaps and jibes without redress or retaliation. She submitted to this indignity, ever tolerant, like her father. But not like Gerard. She was chatty, covering every aspect of her life experience of interaction with others. Schools and mean girls featured. She sang to me, a song she composed for her father, a very long, meandering affair. Yet she stayed with me only long enough for Gerard to finish showering, and then she shadowed him, forsaking all other comforts and entertainments. She missed Gerard with palpable angst, not understanding why one parent had been swapped out for another, one father for another.

Lee, the youngest, was an ever-moving target. Her mother introduced her with the indictment that she was a hooligan like me, her Nana. With tousled curls like Gerard, she outran, outspoke, outwitted all of us. It took her all of five minutes to lay claim to me as her personal property, shoving her older sister off the bed with, 'She's MY nana.'

When Lee was told of her father's death, she turned to her mother. 'Is Nana dead too?'

Later, I sat scrolling on the iPad. Along came ABBA, music Gerard had heard growing up. His favourite 'Fernando' played. My heart went tight as an over-coiled spring. I had 33 percents on the iPad. But I just couldn't, recharge, re-hear… re-member. Not that, and not all those songs Gerard introduced me to, meandering into my room, flicking my computer screen aside to share a song. A song for me to enjoy with him. A song I never knew I loved or needed until then.

Fare thee well

Gone

When I found him lifeless, Gerard had one foot out the window – a childhood habit. I screamed his name, calling him back, begging to go back in time.

I phoned 000. 'My son is dead.'

They wanted more information. There was none to give.

'Pull him off the bed and start CPR,' said the responder.

'It's too late,' I said, but I counted along with her as she followed protocol. I placed my hand gently over Gerard's heart and counted one … two … three …

When the ambulance officers arrived, they were quick to shake their heads, reveal their own sadness, and leave.

I took Gerard's glasses off. I would never see his hazel eyes again, those eyes so like mine.

I phoned Bronson, beautiful, alive Bronson, who would now bend and break. The sight of Bronson's anguish was nearly worse than the shock of Gerard's inert body. My precious Bronson, who had never given up on me, never "voted me off the island", no matter how I failed him. The son who fought and argued for understanding.

The son who said, 'See me. Hear me. Know me,' and then forgave me when I got it wrong, apologised when he got it wrong.

His pain had begun, and I would bear witness to it, thinking I had answers for him but not knowing whether I would get it right.

I once told Bronson that I felt like a parachutist that landed on a church spire instead of the X on the field where I wanted to be, describing how I felt about communicating with him. Understanding him.

Bronson came with Bella, who instinctively brought her calm presence to bear. She sat with us, mourned with us and put her own feelings on hold in order to be there for us. I once said to Bella, 'No matter how pissed off Bronson is with me, you never change towards me.'

Bella smiled, waved a hand towards a corner of the room and said, 'That's over there. It's not mine.'

Bronson became a new kind of man that night.

Two police officers came, a young constable and an older detective. Both needed to interview me.

The young constable went first. He sat opposite the three of us, while the detective sat at the dining table.

The young officer began asking questions, and I answered them. I couldn't tell you one of the questions, or one word I said, other than 'you're a lovely man' every now and then. He was kind, in a way he didn't have to be.

'Mum, don't do that,' said Bronson, embarrassed by my praise.

'Not everyone would do what he is doing with such grace, Bronson. Life is about telling people how you feel at the time, rather than wishing you could tell them when it's too late.'

The questions continued.

'Oh dear,' I said, 'I phoned 911, not 000.'

'Too much American television,' said the detective.

The young officer put his pen down.

I turned to look at the detective.

'I'm good, love. I reckon you've covered everything I need to know,' he said, with a wide smile.

Bronson smiled. 'Yeah, that's Mum.'

A few months later, Bronson told me that he had come across the young officer and was able to tell him how he felt about his care of us. How much it meant to him personally.

'Glad I got that closure,' Bronson said.

Gerard blamed no one in the suicide letter he left for us. 'I'm going home to God,' he said, 'to heal this broken child.'

I'm glad he had peace. I'm glad for his faith. But it is no comfort to me. God is anathema to me.

I wrote verse. Bronson, after reading it, said it was great but too depressing and dark to share at a public memorial, so he wrote the eulogy, a hopeful, beautiful piece in elegant prose.

I gave the Lutheran minister Gerard's teddy bear and Akubra hat to place at the front of the church on the day of the memorial. It was the only useful thing I did that day.

I watched the scattering of Heath Ledger's ashes, and thought at the time that it was beautiful. But. I can't do it. Yet.

I didn't sleep that first night after Gerard died. I don't think I closed my eyes. Bronson and Bella had been with me through the day. I climbed into bed. Mr Clooney lay on the bottom of the bed, facing the doorway as if guarding for intruders.

I held Gerard's coat, the colourful hippy one, cried and said, 'Come back.'

When Bronson arrived in the morning, he was shocked at my appearance.

'Mum, did you sleep?' he asked.

'I was too scared to sleep. Too…' I threw my arms up.

'You look like you belong in the morgue too, Mum. I don't want to lose you, too,' he said, sending me to bed to sleep. And while there, I thought about how I never wanted to worry Bronson again. Never wanted to be the one to put pain in his eyes. Never wanted to see my pain reflected in his eyes.

I would not become a burden. A nuisance, maybe, but not a burden.

The day before, Gerard had wanted the car. A friend had arrived to vent about her daughter, so I didn't notice Gerard's exact comings and goings.

Gerard sourced a Will Kit from a nearby post office, had it witnessed and signed. He seemed a bit busy. He had bought photo albums for each of his children. I had been with him. He chose carefully. If it was a sign, I didn't recognise it as such.

Gerard came to me with the albums and the pile of photos he had printed at Big W. He had slotted the photos into the book, but in one of the books, they were upside down, and he couldn't make his fingers work. So we sat at the table, and I put them the right way up. Gerard watched me with quiet admiration and gratitude.

Gerard had changed all his passwords to the same one. He had sorted everything he owed. At the bottom of the note he left, he had his pin number for his bank debit card, which was lined up on his desk.

He had carefully boxed some favourite things he wanted his brother to have.

I didn't see any of this at first. Didn't see the note. Didn't see the room. I only saw my son. Asleep, but not asleep. There, but gone.

The long life he wished for the rest of us seemed like a death sentence.

The fact that he saw death as the end of his problems, the path of peace, chilled me. This was no knee-jerk reaction. It was an organised plan where he believed we would move on and be better without him.

Did the physical ailments he faced feature in his thinking? I don't know. He had problematic wisdom teeth and couldn't face injections. He fainted when blood was taken unless he was already lying down. He feared the dentist's chair. He took regular pain meds for those aching teeth. He had tried to find out about a general anaesthetic, but that was prohibitive. He was born with strabismus. He suffered from psoriasis and was told he had a high chance of psoriatic arthritis. He had an unpredictable remission from Graves ' disease.

When he first felt the weakening of his muscles, he sought advice from his GP and lowered the doses of any medications that would stultify or sedate, but the weakness and poor balance continued. He had once carried a fridge by himself, but now struggled with jars and lids and turned to me to open the Vegemite and jam jars. It broke my heart.

Did the provisional diagnosis of Motor Neurone Disease play a part in his thinking? I don't know. In the note, he only spoke of love and escape from brokenness.

I didn't see much of him the day before with his errands and the distressed friend who visited me, so that night I felt a pall of sadness that I couldn't explain. I had missed him. I went into his room after he had gone to bed. I placed a hand on either side of his face and said, 'I love you so very much.' This was something I hadn't done since his childhood.

'I love you very much too, Mum.' I kissed his forehead, and rather than move away, he closed his eyes and smiled.

It's all about me now

In the days after Gerard died, I broke a front tooth on Cornflakes. A visit to the dentist seemed like a mountain I couldn't climb, but the sharp edges of the tooth spurred me on to. On reversing at the dental clinic, I backed into the neighbouring fence.

The dentist remarked on it when I finally sat in the chair.

'Oh, dear Lord,' I said, 'did you see that?'

'Everyone saw it,' he said, with the hint of a smile. His nurse nodded.

'Shoot me now,' I said, as I slumped in the chair, thinking of the expense of repairing a fence. The car could wait.

'Don't worry,' said the dentist. 'We've been trying to get that old bloke to take down that derelict fence for years. You should have knocked the thing over, done us a favour.'

'Next time,' I said, relieved.

Every night, I hugged myself at the edge of the bed, whispering, 'Come back, Gerard, come back.'

Every morning, the morning light took me from a dream world where Gerard existed to a dense fog where he did not exist.

With leaden feet, I rose to feed the cat, who was blissfully normal about being a cat.

My nursing friends from my training days phoned, as they had for decades of our lives, knowing instinctively what to say, how to be. It was a bridge. It was sanity in a world that had stopped making sense. They phoned to cheer me up. They phoned for me to cheer them up, restoring my place in the world. We told each other stories, lived in each other's worlds.

I walked in a world where my knowledge and experience of it didn't extend beyond a soughing breath, beyond a hand's breadth, beyond the corner store, beyond the post office where I was forced to collect the mail because we didn't have letterboxes.

Partway through my Honours thesis, I studied and wrote. The thesis examined the connection between poetry and writing about trauma. I found the work oddly therapeutic. There was a way to articulate my grief in fractured verse.

I painted the house. I painted the benches. These were things I would normally have done, but something was shifting.

I missed Gerard like a punch in the chest.

I missed my grandbabies.

I missed my hometown. I missed my father. I missed my childhood. I missed my living son. A son I wanted to cling to like a life raft. A son who was struggling in his own way to find meaning in a dark new world.

I missed the "me" I used to be, the one who woke up with a new way to be useful to the ones I loved, useful to myself. I was no longer needed. I was no longer an advocate.

I missed my friends in NSW.

I missed every damned thing I ever treasured and lost.

The Akubra

Bella, Bronson and I spent the days of the next week together at my place. They went home to their place at night. We talked of a memorial of some kind. Someone suggested a Lutheran minister. He came and sat with us. His visit was marvellous.

Bronson read some verse I had written, only for myself, because that's what I do in life. Put my heart on white pages.

Bronson said it was beautiful but too dark for a service.

'I know,' I said.

Bronson wrote the eulogy. Bella made a magnificent slide show. Gerard's friend Cindy from the local takeaway organised a wake with finger food. Gerard's father paid for the cremation.

What did I do? I don't remember, other than getting up, placing one foot after the other, having conversations where I was not really present.

It took a while after Gerard died for me to sort his clothes and take them to charity shops. I sold a few things. I kept his hippy coat and his red toothbrush.

I put the huge Akubra hat on the Facebook marketplace. It would be difficult to find someone with a head that size, but I received a gentle, tentative enquiry from a guy who confessed that he had dreamed of having an Akubra.

I gave him my address. He arrived at sunset. What a gentle soul he was. I invited him in, but he shook his head.

'I don't like to intrude,' he said, in exactly the way Gerard would have done. 'I don't like to make a woman feel uncomfortable.'

I smiled as he told me his story. He had a group of mates that he went camping with. All the other blokes had Akubras, but he couldn't afford one and felt a bit of a povvo with his old khaki fishing hat. A brand-new Akubra would mean he would finally fit in with the others, not be ashamed or embarrassed on camping trips, do what he loved with friends, and enjoy companionship.

I didn't tell him of the origins of the hat, and he didn't ask.

He handled the hat with reverence, turning it in his hands before putting it on his head. He stroked his unkempt beard. I asked if he wanted a mirror.

'It's fine,' he said, 'it fits as if it was made for me.'

He left the hat on as he handed over the money.

'I can't thank you enough,' he said, as he slowly removed the hat and stared at it.

'Oh, but you have,' I said, 'that's thanks enough and then some.'

He drove down the road into the darkness. The sun had set while we were talking.

I often think of Gerard's Akubra, off camping, getting grubby with life experiences, falling in rivers and being retrieved, sitting in pride of place on the dashboard of a gentle man's AWD, travelling, having the adventures Gerard never had. It makes me smile.

Not good at funerals

You arrive with your sympathy, your desire to console. However, I wish I could convey to you the abrasiveness of your comfort, its sandpaper burden as it scrapes across my bruised heart. A heart that doesn't understand the necessity to beat, wonders why it continues its lub-lub rhythm in spite of its destitution. You crowd and clutter me with your expectations, your desire for my co-operation on one of the worst days of my life.

Sit with me. I'm not good at funerals.

People say stupid stuff, like "they mean well" as if assumed intentions negate my need to defend my fragile grieving soul with solitude. I have no right words for you no matter how long you wait, depending on my resilient responses. I have none of those.

Sit with me. I'm not good at funerals.

While grieving I am trapped, going blindly along, constrained to provide forced gratitude for the ministrations of others who scrape sharp steel chairs across the bare floors of my pain, my foggy vulnerability while I struggle to remember when I last ate, while I forget to lock doors, turn ovens off, while laying my head on a pillow seems like a dark dream to avoid. For if I sleep, I will dream and in that dream my beloved will live and breathe, laugh, listen and live. I can't afford that mythology. I have to write lists. Contact government departments. Converse with coroners and undertakers. Make arrangements with banks. Deal with mail. Make decisions with a mind that no longer holds reason.

Sit with me. I'm not good at funerals.

I am bereft. I do not need the brutality of holding polite conversation, catering to your need for my hospitality. Against my will, I have left the building. The tyranny of your succour is delaying the time when I can sit with my loss without the need to compose the correct responses.

Giving me a list of things to do – things that are expected at funerals is a tyranny, an expectation that stumbles across the field of my peace-need, abrasing the quiet contemplative sanctuary that I am unable to inhabit. You have intruded upon what I really need. A quiet, soft place where I can accomplish those irksome tasks that require a calm uncluttered mind. Allow me to do that while you attend to some mundane task that everyday life requires.

Sit with me. I'm not good at funerals.

I'm dealing with an obscenity. I'm the pawn of a cruel world. I won't make sense. Nothing makes sense. Calling me back to society's expectations of my performative value is not a call that I will answer. I won't read scripture. I won't sing a hymn. I won't "say a few words". That's your need, not mine. Let others observe their own rituals and comforts. I don't share those. They're yours, not mine. Trust me. I will return. But for now…

Sit with me. I'm not good at funerals.

At a memorial someone said, 'Linda's not good at funerals" when I was happy for another to read a poem I had written. This disparaging remark, aimed to remind me of my duty, did not hit its mark. I'm not supposed to be "good at funerals". Arriving to do what you think is best is not the nobility you think it is. The best thing anyone ever did for me when my baby died, was to walk in the door, sit down and entertain my toddler by playing with blocks.

Ask. Ask what is needed, wanted, desired. And if the response is, 'I need you to leave me alone. Come back when I'm sane' then respond with grace. Make a sandwich. Sweep a floor. Lock the doors. Check the oven.

Sit with me. I'm not good at funerals.

The eulogy by Bronson

Dear Gerrard,

You have meant everything to us.

There are no words to express how heartbroken we are, we ache from your loss.

You need not be sorry for leaving us, you fought as long and hard as you could to keep your family loved, safe and happy.

You have shown us an incredible amount of love, kindness, courage and strength that we will carry with us for the rest of our lives.

You taught us so much about life and love and you continue to teach us through your loss the immeasurable value of our own lives and the lives of our loved ones.

You showed through your life that you would want more than anything for us to be happy.

So we will carry on through this pain, and live to honour you and make you proud of how we live our lives. To love and protect each other as you have loved and protected us.

You carried your mother for kilometres up the mountain to safety when you were just a teenager and around the same age stood in the doorway to protect your little brother from violence. Your life is full of examples of what we would call heroism.

And even your final hours are full of examples of selflessness, kindness and love to ease our pain.

We hope and pray more than anything in the world that we will see you again.

Without armour

I am without armour; living my life on the outside of my skin.

It's a hard day, today. I shouldn't write on a hard day. I should write on a better day, a more pulled-myself-together day, but then, perhaps I should write on whatever day I'm having so I'm writing today.

My son Gerard took his own life on July 9, 2019.

He sorted all his things, leaving the least amount of pain he could. He left a letter, 'Sorry Mum, then his children's names … in order.

He blamed no one, ending with, 'I'm going home, where God can heal his broken child.'

I cannot tell you how much I miss him. I miss him with every breath.

All his life he wanted to be a hero to his family. That doesn't mean he was a hero in suicide, undertaking a heroic act. It doesn't mean he left me, though God knows I could argue that point a thousand different ways. He left his life. He left himself.

I'm angry at times. Yesterday I drove past Krispy Cremes, bawled like a baby and said, 'You'll never have another Krispy Crème, did you think of that, you silly boy?'

Yet all the meanings of my heart are best summed up with 'How do I go on without one of the brightest lights of my life?'

After his wife left with his three children he attempted suicide, then, after talking his way out of the mental health unit he messaged me with his usual sparsity of words: "u there mum?"

He arrived off the plane in Op Shop clothes with a suitcase of tattered childhood mementos and a few of his children's' toys that had been left behind in the empty house.

Gerrard was introverted, thoughtful, deep, flawed. Shadowed by inner pain, not tormented by inner demons. He had been living with me, struggling and falling. He turned everything inward, a lifetime habit.

Gerrard had been with me for nearly three years.

I was always afraid. I'd been afraid throughout His father's suicide events, and feared…

I became more afraid as the lawyers bartered.

This for that, 3 days access bargained down to three hours (with 30 days notice) by a pert young thing with trendy, blonde bi-tresses and a legal resume that read like an online dating profile who spelled her name in court in case the judge was senile. B. U. R. N. S.

An intense young father with his lists, dates, papers and facts quiet serious demeanour and precise, quiet words couldn't compete with fast fancy footwork.

Morning Gerard

We always left the "good" out of our morning greetings.

Some might say that talking to the dead is irrational, but death is irrational, and loss is irrational. I guess talking to you is irrational for me. It's not a letter you'll ever receive, words you'll ever hear.

It's a weird thing. The whole business. When you're down and troubled, it's as if every regret, every angst, every past woe gets the mad idea that there's going to be a party in your head, so they round up all the usual suspects, thoughts, and buried nonsense; stuff you've dealt with, bagged, and filed. And then they turn up like a chatty horde of minions, making it impossible for grief to be a solo act. So often, grief is a collection of sorrows, doubts, and fears, many of which belong in the past but want to make an appearance in the present.

Yesterday, or some day before today (the days wander and meander across my life instead of the other way around), I found the songs you bookmarked on my computer. From all the times you interrupted my serious business, flicked my screen aside and played a song you wanted me to hear. With that knowing cheeky smile that said, 'come on, I've always been the boss of you'.

I haven't listened to those songs all the way to the end. I haven't listened to a whole song since you died. Not the Amazing Graces, the Bring Him Homes, not even my pop favourites, Elton, Meatloaf or Jimmy Barnes.

You see, the day you died was the day the music died.

I didn't know you'd bookmarked them when you played them, but then you've always been a sneaky bugger, leaving notes, waking me up by wriggling the whole bed.

Remember the time they sent a box of chocolates home from the school, and we ate them all, alarming your younger brother, who protested, 'The school said we had to…,' to which we laughed and laughed and said how silly it was to send candy home for children to doorknock complete random strangers. Then he ate the chocolates with us. His first lesson in the judiciary.

Three years. Three years without you. And still, that week last month was hell. That anniversary. What a dumb word.

Last night I was in bed watching a cat video. Yes, I know. Then I relaxed and let the videos feed just roll, flicking past nonsense fake stories, laughing at Graham Norton's jokes and listening to bits and pieces of songs. Until I came to one that I didn't want to flick past.

I listened the whole way through. I didn't flick past. It was the perfect song. Irrational, nonsensical, but resonating with beauty in its harmonies and incomprehensible lyrics.

It was The Day the Music Died.

Bureaucracy

The undertakers took Gerard to the Coroner's, whatever and wherever that meant.

He was returned to Gawler to the undertaker's offices. They phoned me and told me that I had to identify him before the cremation.

I shrank within.

I drove slowly and carefully to the undertaker's. Afraid to forget where I was, which road to take, although familiar. I parked miles from other cars. Other objects to graze or hit. I gave way to every vehicle and person I encountered.

I placed a hand on Gerard's chest, gently, softly, as if he was still there, still mine, sleeping, able to feel my touch.

The woman from the undertaker's asked me if I had any clothes that I wanted to bring.

'No,' I said, 'a shroud will do. Like the one there now. Gerard would like that.'

I thought of all the clothes he had rejected. How little he cared for fashion or style. He would rather a shroud, like the Christ he loved and with whom he so desperately wished a reunion.

After the cremation, I had to return to pick up the ashes.

I carried the polished timber box on my hip, the way I had carried Gerard as a babe. Like Gerard, the box was heavier than I expected. I shifted it from one hip to the other.

Forty-two years after bringing my son home from the hospital, I was bringing his ashes home.

At home, by the fire, while Mr Clooney the cat snored loudly, I just sat, holding that polished timber box, and singing a mish-mashed lullaby because I could never remember the words.

I forgive you

it's okay
I forgave you
in the very first moment.

Here's looking at you kid

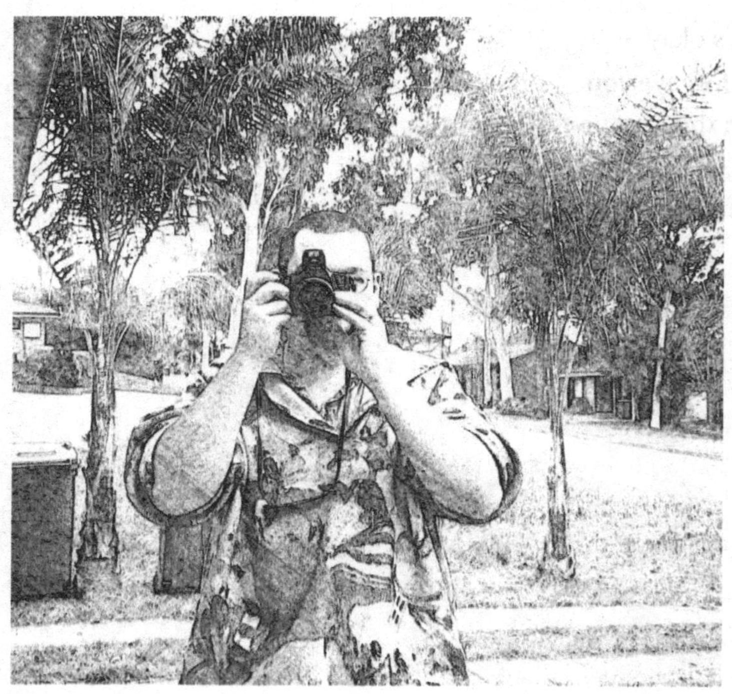

To accept, to understand, to celebrate

I wish someone had told me earlier that my son had autism.

I wish someone had told me he was locked into a world he didn't choose; a world I didn't cause.

I wish someone had told me I didn't need to rescue him, or force him out of his narrow prison.

I wish someone had told me that all I had to do was join him in his world, sit there with him while he found the courage and acceptance to find his own way into the world that judged him odd; different.

I wish someone had told me how easy it would be to celebrate him when I understood.

Autism

Defining autism: Tony Attwood

Professor Tony Attwood is well known for his advocacy and treatment of autistic children and adults and for sharing his knowledge in seminars and podcasts. He has an Honours degree in Psychology from the University of Hull, Masters Degree in Clinical Psychology from the University of Surrey and a PhD from the University of London.

According to Attwood, children and adults with autism have a **different, not defective**, way of thinking. Contrary to historic perceptions of autism, research proposes that the cause is not due to emotional deprivation or failure of parental bonding. High-functioning children and adults have typical intellectual abilities but display unique behaviours and responses from early childhood.

Professionals and service agencies tend to see children and adults with problems that are conspicuous and difficult to treat or resolve, which may lead to an overly pessimistic view of long-term outcomes. The autistic person typically learns to improve their ability to socialise, converse, and understand others' thoughts and feelings.

They learn to express their feelings, overcoming their earlier struggles, which Attwood describes as 'completing a jigsaw puzzle of several thousand pieces without a picture on the box'.

Further explanation

There is impaired social interaction, which may be less evident when the person is engaged in an activity of interest or feels comfortable. Autistic people struggle to interpret the facial expressions of others and may prefer conversations where they are not required to hold eye contact.

There is difficulty understanding the expectations and "rules" of society. This is evident regardless of cultural or racial heritage. Social expectations are often misunderstood and sometimes resisted or refused. Social anxiety is often present. Pressure to conform may be met with distress or anger, suggesting discomfort rather than rebellion. They experience physical and emotional exhaustion from socialising.

They have difficulty with conversational skills and perceive small talk as annoying. Conviction and inflexibility in their worldview often make them appear to be talking down to others. There may be differences in speech inflexion, patterns and use of language. They tend to make literal interpretations.

In close relationships, autistics may struggle with expressing their degree of love in a way expected by others, deeming constant reassurance unnecessary. They struggle with the concept of reciprocating with others and with the usual actions of empathy.

When it comes to making friends, autistic individuals may prefer the company of older or younger people rather than that of people their own age or at the same developmental level.

Special interests are present at an early age. Autistic individuals frequently have intense, focused interests where much of the knowledge gained is self-directed and self-taught. The special interest serves as a means of pleasure, learning, self-concept, and confidence, which parents, teachers, and therapists can utilise in positive ways. It is essential to recognise that special interests benefit both individuals with autism and society as a whole. The special interest helps reduce anxiety and offers relaxation from social and societal pressures.

They are perceived as blunt, brutally honest or rude. They value direct, unambiguous communication and conversation. They exhibit a strong sense of justice for themselves and others. They value loyalty. They have a distinctive sense of humour. They may prefer solitude over company and spurn crowded, noisy events unless in the area of their interest.

When it comes to getting things done, autistic individuals often struggle to cultivate effective organisational skills and time-management abilities. They value routine, certainty, and predictability.

Sensitivity to sound, light, and touch can lead to sensory overload and increased stress. Sensitivity usually involves particular sounds, but can also extend to touch, light, food taste and texture, or certain aromas. Children may respond too strongly or not strongly enough to pain and discomfort.

Those with sensory sensitivity often become hypervigilant, tense, and easily distracted in environments with lots of sensory stimulation, such as classrooms. Indicators are typically more pronounced during early childhood, though they may persist as enduring traits in certain adults.

Motor coordination difficulties are frequently observed.

Autistic people strongly pursue knowledge, truth, and fairness. They might be more concerned with finding solutions to problems than with meeting others' social or emotional needs. Creativity and results are prioritised over teamwork. Meticulous attention to detail ensures errors are promptly identified.

The gender dynamic

Autistic females often display traits that differ from those seen in males. Many autistic girls remain undiagnosed because the signs of autism are less obvious than in boys. A girl with autism may hide her uncertainty during social interactions with peers, relying on imitation and performance. She is likely to be well-behaved and less disruptive at school, and so is less likely to be noticed. Missing an early diagnosis delays intervention and support, and can cause autistic girls to feel defective, increasing the risk of mental health issues in adolescence.

A summary

A different, not defective, way of thinking.
a strong desire for knowledge, truth and perfection.
There is a different perception of personal and social situations.
There is a difference in sensory experiences.
Motor clumsiness, problems with handwriting.
Hypersensitivity to specific auditory and tactile experiences
Problems with organisational and time management skills
Unusual speech patterns and language
Restrictive interests, unusual in intensity and focus.
Preference for routine and consistency.
Priority to problem-solve rather than meet expectations.
Challenges in teamwork or collaboration.
preferring to work alone.
They may perceive errors not apparent to others.
Exhibit attention to detail, rather than noticing the big picture.
Direct, honest, may be considered disrespectful and rude.·
They are determined and have a strong sense of social justice.
The person may actively seek and enjoy solitude.
They value loyalty in personal and professional relationships.
They have a distinct sense of humour.
Difficulty with management and expression of emotions.
They may have high levels of anxiety, sadness or anger.
Difficulty expressing the expected degree of love and affection.
A tendency to make a literal interpretation of what is said,
Delay developing compromise and conflict resolution.·
Use of intelligence rather than intuition with social information
Physical and emotional exhaustion from socialising.

Factors that contribute to positive outcomes:

Early diagnosis.·
Acceptance of the diagnosis.·
Emotional and practical support.
Relationship with a mentor.
Acquiring further knowledge through personal research.
Achieving success in a workplace or a particular area of interest.
Redesigning the environment to fit with needs and sensitivities.
Accepting their uniqueness, potential and limitations.
No longer seeking to become someone they cannot be. ·

Numerous autistic adults say that as they matured, they gained an intellectual understanding of social interactions, which often led to successful integration into social settings. Noticeable symptoms of autism may become less apparent as time goes on, and some progress to a point where only subtle differences and difficulties remain. The person has progressed beyond a diagnostic category, and the term 'lifelong eccentricity' is more appropriate.

Tony Attwood states: "I have valued friends and relatives with Autism. I see people with autism as a bright thread in the rich tapestry of life. Our civilisation would be extremely dull and sterile if we did not have and treasure people with autism."

A psychiatrist: Dr Jay

Attentive listening without judgment gives both children and adults the freedom and space to experience their thoughts and feelings. It also creates a comfortable environment, encouraging them to express and reveal their emotions. Quiet, attentive listening allows careful observation and assists thoughtful diagnosis.

Clinical observation is essential for a diagnosis of autism. Due to the varying severity of autism symptoms, a thorough diagnosis will take time and require careful observation of the patient, as well as careful listening to the behaviours reported by parents, teachers and others involved in their care.

Practitioners are seeing more patients with autism because of increased awareness of this disorder. They are also seeing them earlier, often as young as three years of age. Children are often referred by teachers who observe the child's obsessive behaviours; for example, a child may be unable to put aside their spelling class work and move on to the next activity due to a compulsive need to finish, or may find they are unable to progress to the next maths question because they have not completed the previous one in an examination. This causes significant distress and anxiety. Teachers also see that some children simply do not understand the rules, and they may act inappropriately socially. The child who isolates socially may have ongoing difficulties. I have seen the benefit of increased teacher awareness of autism.

Children with autism often appear immature compared with their peers. They exhibit delays because their social interpretation and expression are impaired. Learning is an interactive activity, and children with autism lack relational skills. As the child matures, the presentation of symptoms changes. A nurturing and supportive environment, or its absence, has a significant impact on their personality development. Sometimes children learn to model appropriate behaviours, such as looking someone directly in the eye, which increases their comfort with others and their level of social acceptance. Disturbances in their social interactions inhibit their engagement with their social group and classmates.

Practitioners also see older patients who were not previously diagnosed with autism. These older patients may have experienced depression or been perceived as eccentric. They have a history of struggling to obtain employment and to engage in relationships with others. As with children, the incidence is typically higher in males. Autism has existed for some time, but many people have been undiagnosed and often overlooked due to a lack of information.

There is a significant difference between those who have received effective treatment and those who have not. Intervention, acceptance and understanding play a significant role in the development of people with autism. When they feel supported and connected to their environment, their functioning level increases dramatically. A positive environment cannot be underestimated for its beneficial effect.

If an autistic person has suffered in their early twenties and been misdiagnosed or misunderstood, the diagnosis can be a liberating light-bulb moment. For some, the diagnosis is all they need.

They haven't been searching for excuses in life, but for an explanation. The autism diagnosis can be an enlightening and gratifying reason to accept their individuality and seek situations and relationships that suit them, rather than ones that cause discomfort and anxiety.

When it comes to community support and treatment, a diagnosis empowers self-advocacy and access to services and resources for education, employment, social interaction, and mental health. A diagnosis can do all this and restore dignity to a late-diagnosed adult autistic person.

Adult diagnosis is better than ignorance. Late diagnosis means lost time. Time that could have illuminated difficulties, brought acceptance, and led to more appropriate paths for the future. Diagnosis is invaluable. It brings understanding. Essentially, it is a map of the individual, describing who they are.

Late diagnosis is more likely among high-functioning autistic adults than among those with a more pronounced autistic profile, as developmental delays and more prominent behaviours are not as evident.

Being diagnosed as autistic as an adult is a confronting experience. So many people have suffered from incorrect diagnoses and treatment that there is often acute relief once they realise they are different. Their childhood history often points to a self-contained childhood. They may have been described as old souls, quirky, withdrawn, or anxious about changes in routine or new situations, especially when those situations involve meeting people.

As we saw previously, they also find their workmates social

behaviours confusing because they struggle to interpret the workplace's social constructs. They don't play social games, and their brutal honesty and sense of justice may offend.

Another area that prompts an autistic adult to seek treatment or therapy is difficulty connecting and forming strong romantic relationships. Their difficulty adapting and compromising inhibits their ability to work together peacefully in a relationship. They usually have difficulty understanding a partner's desire for reassurance.

My child is autistic.

Autistic adults are often confronted with their uniqueness at the time of their child's diagnosis. They may then see parallels, identify with their children, and seek help, or fiercely deny their own tendencies and their child's difficulties. If a parent finds that their child's profile resonates with them personally, they can become not only more informed about themselves but also about their child, and become their child's most valuable asset.

In creating change for their child, they can foster their own acceptance and claim their unique abilities and the right to be different. It's not uncommon for the autistic adult to find others with autism at this time, and the connection can be empowering. The sense of release from conforming to society's narrow boundaries can help them build self-esteem and form true friendships.

Strange as it may seem, the internet often helps autistic people relate and connect without the stress of interpreting facial expressions, jokes, sarcasm, and innuendo. They can find others with similar interests and communicate freely.

You don't have autism. Who told you that?

Undermining a carefully considered diagnosis has a negative impact on the autistic person. Statements like 'Who says you have that? You don't seem to have that. I have a nephew, cousin, relative, or friend with that, and you're not like them at all.' These pressures are added to the pressure on the person to perform at a socially acceptable level that is deemed normal. It diminishes the perception of someone's intelligence.

Many people assume that all neurodivergent people look different, believing they "walk funny, talk funny, don't smile, and do weird stuff". This attitude of personal, professional or social discrimination affects not only the neurodivergent person but also those closest to them. "Protecting" someone from a diagnosis enables the crippling narrowness of the autistic person's life to continue, unchallenged and misunderstood. Their future remains constricted and unfulfilled.

Autistic people can also vehemently reject a diagnosis. One of the saddest things in this situation is that the autistic person themselves may reject anyone who disagrees or tries to point them to the source of their distress and disconnection. They can perceive disagreement as betrayal. How can they trust someone who doesn't see life the way they do? The old description of autism as "failure of mother to bond with infant" is not only outdated but also categorically false.

Social discomfort levels lead autistic adults to seek to avoid social interaction, especially in groups. They may exhibit stony silence, excessive or minimal grooming, blunt answers to questions, closed body language, withdrawal and growing isolation.

These are not behaviours intended to attract attention, cause trouble, play or delude; they are adopted to protect. Often, an autistic person would rather sit one-on-one with a friend or stay home with family. All kinds of social gatherings make little sense to them. This may sound very much like an introspective, reserved personality, but whereas a shy person may prefer limited interaction, an autistic person needs it.

However, it would be wrong to assume that all autistic people are antisocial. People on the spectrum desire interaction. Isolation does not bring satisfaction or contentment. Retreating from discomfort is different from seeking solitude.

It is important to understand that autistic people do not lack any emotions in their emotional landscape. They do, however, experience difficulty in articulating their emotions in a way that satisfies others. They are constantly struggling to deal with people who 'don't say what they mean'.

Studies indicate an increased incidence of substance abuse and criminality among children with ADHD who do not receive medication as they become adults. Untreated autism in children leads to increased vulnerability and impaired social functioning in adulthood. One should not underestimate the ongoing suffering of families and patients with this developmental delay.

Medication is not prescribed merely to control behaviours but to assist with the cognitive delays associated with this disorder (information-processing delays rather than intelligence) and the significant anxiety, depression and hopelessness that can arise. No one would deny medication to a child with a brain disorder causing seizures, yet there remains considerable emotional debate about treating the obsessive behaviours and crippling anxiety of autism, as well as the distressing symptoms of ADHD.

Medication doesn't change the world. It manages a problem. Mental conditions deserve the same respect as physical ones, and medication, when carefully prescribed and monitored, can have significant benefits for mental illness.

Nor does medication have to be ongoing or permanent. It is often a bridging strategy that helps a confused, disordered mind attain the peace needed to concentrate and effect change in their lives. A good psychiatrist is essential, as no amount of therapy or intervention can replace a psychiatrist's medical training and clinical experience.

There is always a concern that an adolescent or young adult will seek to 'feel normal' by self-medicating with illegal drugs or alcohol, which can create a vicious cycle of depression and anxiety.

Be careful before you refuse the option. Medications are uniquely designed.

The medication of choice for autism is antipsychotic therapy. It is not desirable to sedate or slow the person's thinking, or to alter mood.

Sometimes the main benefit of medication for an autistic person is that it fosters a calm state of mind, where the person can reason, connect cause and effect, and think ahead, projecting the likely outcomes of their behaviour and its consequences.

They are less anxiety-driven and more thought-driven, able to use a reflective reasoning approach that may be impossible when distressed.

This calmer frame of mind may facilitate recognition of the impact of their actions on others, enhance empathic understanding, and promote greater participation in the workforce.

A psychiatrist brings knowledge of sound scientific research, a commitment to evidence-based practice, and an intimate understanding of pharmacology and its effects on the brain. Any body of work, be it a parent's narrative or a manual claiming to be The Answer to all your questions, is unbalanced without the input of the doctors who provide crisis intervention in Accident & Emergency clinics, treat patients in institutions, and care for mentally ill clients across all areas of treatment. An office where consultations occur is only the tip of the iceberg. Most psychiatrists have completed more than 14 years of study, including general medicine.

While much still remains to be learned about human brain functioning, major advances have been made over the last 50 years. Today's psychiatrists have the added benefit of parallel advances in pharmacology and are better trained than ever before.

We cannot ignore the stories of practitioners at the interface of the business end—the dark side—where there are late or missed diagnoses, treatment failures, or self-medication with illegal drugs. We also witness the fallout in the justice system, including courts, prisons, and rehabilitation facilities, where people with mental health issues are represented in large numbers. While many people use mood-altering drugs to enhance social experiences or experience euphoria, an autistic person, or someone with frontal lobe impairment, is more likely to take substances merely to 'feel normal'.

While the autistic person can suffer anxiety and frustration in a world out of kilter and among people who don't seem to understand how things should be, a world they 'don't see eye-to-eye with', a world they believe could easily be changed to fit their reality, if only everyone else could see what needs to be done. It is not that the autistic person's perceptions are skewed, nor that their assessments are faulty. For them, very little time is spent on introspective questioning of 'what did I do wrong' or 'how did I contribute to the problem'. There is little room for doubt on their horizon.

Their spouse, family and friends can feel deep heartache watching their loved one at such odds with the world. Partners, work colleagues and families of autistic people toss and turn at night, trying to understand them and their behaviour. All the while, the autistic person remains immersed in a world of anxiety or discomfort, in a disordered world.

Retreat is self-preservation. For autistic people who struggle to relate to others, the next step is often to limit contact with those who push them out of their comfort zones, and then, gradually, with many others. Many therapists report on the living conditions of severely socially maladapted autistic people. They live in isolation. It's not unusual for them to live in their cars or in tiny, cramped rooms. Anywhere the world doesn't intrude, bring confrontation or conflict. It's all too hard. They desire human interaction, contact and friendship, but their attempts too often fail.

There are so many theories and myths, offers of cures, and things to blame, few of which have any merit; many add panic and a financial burden to an already overwhelmed family. Parents are so stressed and hungry for solutions that a referral from a well-meaning friend, counsellor or family member may not receive the scrutiny it deserves.

Autism is a lifelong developmental disorder that relates to the individual landscape of the frontal lobe. Early intervention is key, and the earlier it occurs, the better the long-term prognosis and outcomes. Any therapy that offers a generalised, i.e., one-size-fits-all, approach is suspect, as is any therapy, vitamin or dietary regime that claims to cure the condition. Accepting the reality of the condition is often the greatest gift to an autistic person.

Therapies must stand the test of science.

No one would undertake every promise offered for the treatment of a physical disease without research, and the same scrutiny needs to be applied to programs, regimes and therapies for autism, and its allied conditions.

A strong genetic link to autism has been proven. Often, in discussions about a recently diagnosed family member, someone in the corner says, 'Old Uncle Ned was like that'. Then there are the silent ones who secretly think—They're talking about me.

Autistic people have always been here. There is no solid evidence that autism is on the rise. Autism has existed as long as there have been humans; we have simply missed the clues. We've been looking right past autistic people for a long time. Past them and through them.

Children often begin to show autistic tendencies before their second birthday. I think it's pertinent to consider that this period of presentation coincides with the age when children are beginning to socialise in a more constructive manner, when general practitioners, teachers, family and friends are measuring or comparing maturation, task ability and age-appropriate skills and behaviour.

It would be a shame to label vaccinations as causative when the relationship may be no more than a coincidence of timing. After all, it is a weighty decision. It's not on a par with deciding whether or not to give your child braces—the diseases a child is vulnerable to without vaccination are potentially fatal. A child with Whooping Cough is heartrending; an epidemic is a tragedy.

Personality is separate from any diagnosis, although it will affect the response and treatment. Autistic people can be extroverted, introverted, cautious, risk-taking, shy, assertive or retiring, just like the rest of us. It is commonly perceived that other conditions piggyback on autism, but the simple fact is that OCD, ADHD, Personality Disorder, Bipolar, and Schizophrenia all exist in the frontal area of the brain. Someone with autism is no more likely to have these other conditions than the average person.

Community awareness about autism has also been fostered by many wonderful autistic characters portrayed in films, with wonderful sensitivity and authenticity. More importantly, they are quirky yet fully developed personalities who are engaging and endearing despite their eccentricities. The series 'Austin' with Michael Theo is a fine example of this.

There is an increase in referrals from General Practitioners and Paediatricians. We would do well to remember that although the term autism has been around for some time, knowledge has been slow to develop. This isn't unusual in any area of medical science. It takes time to learn, research, test and apply.

This is even more relevant when it comes to studies that involve understanding the brain, often referred to as 'the last frontier'. Be proactive, but have patience. There are so many dedicated professionals working towards solutions, seeking answers.

We're learning. One boon that has emerged from recent research is the enlightened concept of an autism spectrum. This has resulted from extensive study across the globe by researchers with no agenda, payout or collective bias. Essentially, Asperger's Syndrome is now part of the Autism Spectrum of conditions, and the DSM V has been updated to reflect the acceptance of Asperger's as being on the autistic continuum. This is an advance in thinking and practice.

A good practitioner will base their assessment on the degree of 'life impact', the level of functioning at work, the level of anxiety and triggers for distress, the ability to relate effectively to family, and the ability to process information. If there is pain, disconnection or disability in these areas, a diagnosis is more than a label.

Tips on dealing with an autistic child.

Give your autistic child clear, concise instructions. One at a time. Make lists. This also applies to men. And most women. Pretty much everyone, when you come to think of it. Well, not teachers; don't give them any instructions, just polite suggestions. And smile a lot. They don't get much of that.

Stay calm and focused with your child.

They won't. Not to start with anyway. Yes, that isn't fair; life isn't fair so get over it. They will respond to calm. Refuse to listen until they talk calmly. This does not work with toddlers, *what does?* Say to them, 'my brain can't work when you are yelling, it scrambles my thoughts and I can't talk to you.' They seem to understand scrambled brain syndromes.

Tackle one issue at a time. Stepwise.

Ignore bad behaviour. This requires the fortitude of a Russian army and deafness would be a bonus. But it works. Withdraw eye contact.

Disengage from conflict.

Don't answer repeated questions when you've already said no. When they say, 'You haven't explained that, I don't understand,' what they are really saying is—'You haven't agreed with me yet, and that isn't good enough.' Remember, with an autistic person, that the argument itself is usually the point. The ability to engage you in the struggle is the goal, and you will howl, weep, rant, explain and lie down wishing for a swift and painless death before they even draw breath.

Don't give in; refuse to enter in.

I locked myself in my room. Apparently, this is less likely to be classified as child abuse than locking the child in. Of course, the worry that they'll destroy the remainder of the house while you're in there takes the edge off any pleasure you get, so just increase your house insurance to cope.

Reward good behaviour.

You may need a microscope for this. But when you do find it, don't just acknowledge it, *celebrate* it. You will be surprised by how driven and thrilled your child will be with simple praise and success. These are very motivated children. You only have to listen to them nag to know they have the tenacity of clams. So don't smash them; pry them open when they are relaxed. Don't try to discuss and lay down the law when they are exhausted. And they are emotionally exhausted a lot, even when their mouths are still going ninety to the dozen with the Blah.

Start as you mean to continue.

Try not to change the rules or the routine once you have laid it down. Even a short detour on a shopping trip feels like trickery and sabotage to an autistic person. If you need to change things, reassure them at the time and discuss later. Say stuff like, 'I know this is hard for you, but I need to do this, and I will only do it in emergencies.' Split shopping or visiting trips; do the team thing where the child is needed, and then drop them off in their comfort zone, continuing the rest yourself. This will make your life easier.

Making your life easier is a valid lifestyle choice.

Remember that your child didn't choose this any more than they chose the colour of their eyes. Remember that they love you. Yes, it is a clinging fearful desperate and suffocating love, but *it is love.*

Allow for the fact that their starting point is often fear. The journey is often seasoned with dread and anxiety but the destination is all the sweeter for this painful beginning. They are warriors in a battle you can't see but in the stillness of the calm times you will begin to understand.

Treat yourself well.

Battle fatigue is as deadly as the battle itself, if not more so. Reward yourself. Don't assume someone else will. No child needs the example of strained martyrdom.

Substitute favourite things, i.e. obsessions. Replace rather than confiscate. Hell hath no fury like an autistic person when their pet rock is taken. Don't take things just because they annoy *you.* Remember anything that says familiar to them says home and that means safe. While Gerard was fond of soft toys, he was never without a complex Lego project, which he would meticulously glue together.

Get expert help when you need it.

Ask questions. Listen. Learn. An ounce of prevention is worth a lifetime of battling and regret. It gets better. Knowledge will set you free. Demand it. Use it. Give it to others even if they don't ask for it. If they are going to judge you with their eloquently raised eyebrows they might as well hear the truth.

'My child has autism, it's not an excuse, it is an explanation.'

At nearly every author talk I give there is at least one mother wrestling with a small child. A child who appears to have the strength of a boa constrictor, the tenacity of a limpet and the energy of a tornado.

When she is able, the woman raises her hand.

'Do they ever leave home?' she asks.

I read her eyes.

They mirror exactly what I felt not so many years ago.

I wrote for all those mothers, fathers, grandparents, family and friends, who agonise like I did over whether this life of chaos is all they will ever know.

I have no wisdom of the ages, no guarantees or promises other than opening the door to my fractured, hopeful life and the gift of saying,

---

'You do not walk alone.'

Mental Health Crisis Support

If you or someone you know is in **immediate danger**, please call **Triple Zero (000)** or go to your nearest **hospital emergency department.**

Australia offers a wide range of mental health services, from 24/7 crisis helplines to specialized support for different communities and life stages

Immediate Crisis Support (24/7)

- Emergency: Call 000
- Lifeline: 13 11 14 (Crisis support)
- Suicide Call Back Service: 1300 659 467
- 13YARN: 13 92 76 (For Aboriginal & Torres Strait Islander people)
- MensLine Australia: 1300 78 99 78 (For men)
- 1800RESPECT: 1800 737 732 (Sexual assault/domestic violence support)
- Kids Helpline: 1800 55 1800 (Ages 5–25)

General & Youth Mental Health Services

- **Beyond Blue:** 1300 22 4636 (Support for anxiety, depression, and suicide prevention)
- **Headspace:** 1800 650 850 (Youth mental health 12-25)
- **SANE Australia:** 1800 187 263 (Specialist support for complex mental health issues)
- **ReachOut:** ReachOut.com (Information and support for young people)
- **Griefline:** 1300 845 745 (Support for loss and grief)

Free Support & Specific Programs

- **Medicare Mental Health Centres:** 1800 595 212 (Free, no referral required)
- **NewAccess (Beyond Blue):** 1300 22 4636 (Free mental health coaching)
- **Brother to Brother:** 1800 435 799 (Crisis support for Aboriginal men)

- **Butterfly Foundation:** 1800 334 673 (Eating disorders)
- **Black Dog Institute:** blackdoginstitute.org.au (Digital tools and apps)

Digital & Information Resources
- Head to Health: headtohealth.gov.au (Government site for finding services)
- WellMob: wellmob.org.au (Aboriginal & Torres Strait Islander online resources)
- eMHprac: emhprac.org.au (Directory of digital mental health resources)

Mental health and suicide prevention contacts

A list of organisations, websites and services that offer support, counselling, research and information about mental health and suicide prevention. https://www.health.gov.au/topics/mental-health-and-suicide-prevention/mental-health-and-suicide-prevention-contacts#:~:text=Lifeline&text=Contact%20Lifeline%20for%20support%20if,contact%20their%20confidential%20online%20chat

For ongoing mental health issues, it is recommended to see a General Practitioner (GP) for a Mental Health Treatment Plan to access Medicare-subsidized sessions with a psychologist.

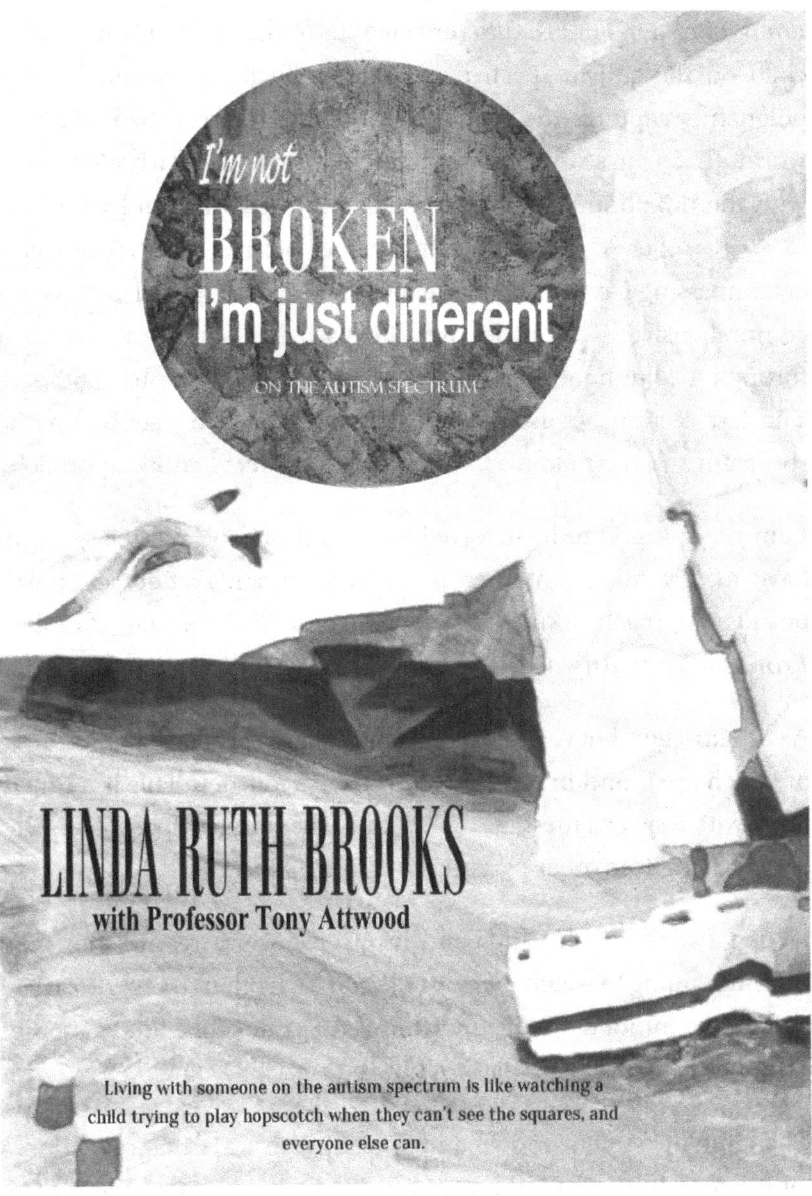

This book is a celebration, a conversation.

I'm not broken, I'm just different takes us to the heart of living with a child on the autism spectrum. In an unflinching account, Brooks poignantly captures the muddled stumbling between two worlds— worlds that seem so desperately different at first. About a boy obsessed with the unfathomable and a mother obsessed with understanding him. A roller coaster ride from the bizarre to the obscene, encompassing the poetic and the hilarious, heartache and joy. Brooks comprehensively chronicles her life with her son from his birth through to adulthood—ending with his fearless flight into manhood. The last section, focuses on the struggles faced by adults on the spectrum and their families with an informative, scientific approach.

I am very pleased to be involved with Linda's book. I think we both have a very important message, and I certainly endorse Linda's positive approach. I know it will change the lives of many families. *Professor Tony Attwood*

As a counsellor, I have discovered a number of special pearls, a couple of which are found in Linda and Bronson's journey. This is a timely book with a special message. Linda and I met for a purpose. I feel this book is her gift to other parents. *Dr Steele Fitchett*

A long-awaited book. Linda and Bronson have a great relationship; it's entertaining to watch them bounce off each other. I once described Linda's parenthood—'You enjoy him; that's one of the finest assets of a mother you offer, regardless of how he reacts.' *Dr Jay*

Changing the system and creating meaning in ways that open doors for others. Throughout, there is an overwhelming sense of gratitude. An inspirational story that will be enjoyed by anyone who has struggled through difficult odds. *Magdalena Ball*

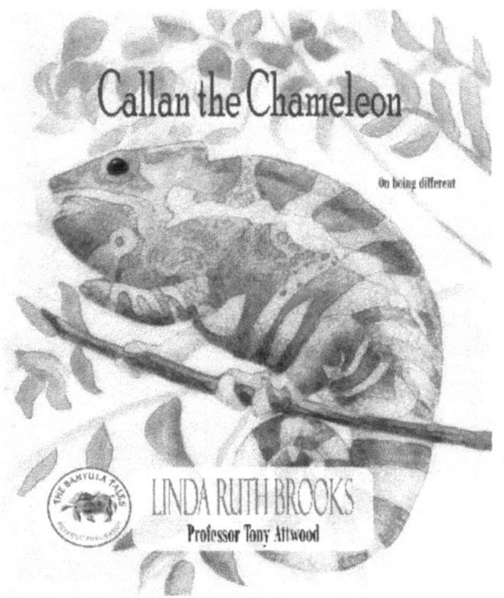

Callan the Chameleon

Callan the Chameleon lived in a tall lilly pilly tree with pink-tipped leaves. The leaves of the lilly pilly tree grow very thick. Callan felt safe in the rustling tree that was home.

The book's theme is the acceptance of our differences.

The main character, Callan, has tendencies that are parallel to Autism Spectrum Disorder. The story addresses this in a subtle way and celebrates our unique personality traits and individual talents. The story revolves around Callan and his bush animal friends, including Emily Echidna, Kyle Koala, Katie Kookaburra, Wesley Wombat, Freya the Frilled-Necked Lizard, and other uniquely Australian animals.